It's **NOT** about

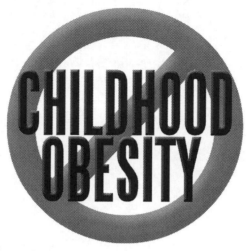

It **IS** about

BEING

HEALTHY

FOR LIFE

Dr. Olga Vaca Durr

Inspiring Voices®

A Service of **Guideposts**

Inspiring Voices books may be ordered through booksellers or by contacting:

Inspiring Voices
1663 Liberty Drive
Bloomington, IN 47403
www.inspiringvoices.com
1-(866) 697-5313

Because of the dynamic nature of the Internet, any web addresses or
links contained in this book may have changed since publication and
may no longer be valid. The views expressed in this work are solely those
of the author and do not necessarily reflect the views of the publisher,
and the publisher hereby disclaims any responsibility for them.

Any people depicted in stock imagery provided by Thinkstock are
models, and such images are being used for illustrative purposes only.

Certain stock imagery © Thinkstock.

ISBN: 978-1-4624-0411-7 (e)
ISBN: 978-1-4624-0412-4 (sc)

Library of Congress Control Number: 2012921160

Printed in the United States of America

Inspiring Voices rev. date:11/08/2012

To Naomi Arriaga Vaca:
Thanks, Momma, for believing I could do things
I never thought I could even reach!

To George E. Peyrot, Jr.:
Thanks, George, for showing me running is not all
that bad!

It's about being healthy for life!

—H4L

Contents

PREFACE

Strangely enough, this book all started at a time when I weighed the most I have ever weighed in my life and was the least healthy. In 2007, I finally went back to college to finish a life goal, one I had started in 1999, but due to "life happening"—as I sometimes refer to it—I had to put my goal on a back burner. Then, in 2007, the back burner finally moved to the forefront of my life, and it was time to get off the fence and make my dreams become a reality. The dream, which was actually ignited by my Momma, was to get a doctorate. Completing a doctorate includes writing a dissertation, a really long paper full of research and statistics, reading a ton of articles, lots of deadlines, working hours on end with not much sleep, and an overabundance of stress. I know, it doesn't sound like anything fun and exciting, but going into the challenge, I looked more at the end result, getting my doctorate, and that was enticing to me, at least enticing enough to dive on in again.

When you start a dissertation, you must have a topic, and usually by the time you finish your coursework, that topic has either been completely changed a few times or whittled down a great deal. From my very first semester, I knew my topic would be childhood obesity; I just was not certain what my variables were going to be. (Variables are used to measure outcomes.) As the journey started, I knew I wanted to do more on the topic and began giving presentations for parents on the topic of childhood obesity, which actually worked well in my job at that time as coordinator for parent and community involvement. For the next three years of college, I researched the topic of childhood obesity, read stories, found information, charts, etc. I finished my coursework one semester late (graduating July 31, 2010) but encountered a huge slough of roadblocks within those three years.

Yet, it was a time during those three years that caused the first spark of this book. In 2009, I was a speaker at a conference, and the title of my session was *Are You Killing Your Kids?* The conference was aimed toward parents, and my session specifically talked about childhood obesity rates and what parents can do to help. After I finished my session, I noticed a mother who had come in at the beginning of the session and was obviously very angry. When she walked in, she had a scowl on her face. She put her feet up on the chair in front of her and sat with her arms folded across her chest throughout the entire session. As the session concluded, I was shocked when she came up to talk to me. She waited until everyone was finished talking to me before she began her conversation, even after I made eye contact with her and asked how she was.

Finally, we had our conversation, which started something like this. She said, "Well, as you can see, I'm fat, my husband is fat, and at home, we have two fat boys." She continued to tell me, "Both my husband's parents and my parents are all fat." Then she asked, "So what do we do?" For me, this was the eye-opening question—when you are fat and your parents are fat, how do you *not* raise fat children? It was then that I realized: if parents do not know how to be healthy, how will they ever be able to teach their children to be healthy?

At that moment, I knew I had to write a book for teenagers, young people, and kids who just wanted to learn how to be healthy for life. As an educator and a former teenager myself, I know firsthand how teens sometimes think our parents do not know the answer. Sometimes we just don't want to listen to what they have to say, only to realize years later that maybe they did know. On the contrary, what if our parents really do not know or do not have all the answers? Then where do you go to find answers and get help? How do you learn to live a healthy life when no one around us knows either?

I refused to allow the slough of roadblocks that were either around me or within me to become my excuse for not finishing my goal and not getting this book written. Even worse, in addition to the slough of roadblocks during these three challenging years, I had gained weight, and my health was on a downhill slide, leading me on the road to obesity, with numerous negative medical effects. So, when I finally walked across that stage to collect the proof that I achieved my goal, my first priority was getting healthy for life and then starting my book, in that order. However, once again life happened. Nevertheless, this time, no more *excuses*. Today I am leading my journey toward being healthy for life, as are my children, my husband, some siblings, and some nieces and nephews!

ACKNOWLEDGMENTS

I would like to express my sincere appreciation and thanks to my husband, children, Daddy, and family members who encouraged my efforts in making this book a reality: thank you for the comments, concern, listening when I needed help, and your support.

Thank you to Dr. J. Austin Vasek for helping complete my first enormous task, which was the research for this book. Also, thank you to Dr. Randy Baca, Dr. Genie Jhnigoor, and Dr. Patti D. Ward for joining me as we completed that task.

Thank you to Jeannette Cannon for her pictures. Check her out on Facebook at jcannonphotography or jeannettecannonart@gmail.

Also, thank you to Jack Pike for his photography. Mr. Pike is a true American Hero, check him out on Facebook at Jack T. F. Pike.

DISCLAIMER

The information provided in *It's Not about Childhood Obesity; It's about Being Healthy for Life!* is intended as a general tool and reference for readers. The author is not rendering professional medical services, and the content is made available with this understanding. Although the author made every effort to provide current and accurate information, readers should be aware that the author accepts no responsibility for the accuracy and completeness of the material in this book and recommends consulting a doctor before making any major dietary or physical changes. Although the purpose of this book is to educate, the author shall have neither liability nor responsibility to any person or entity with respect to any loss or damage caused or suspected to be caused, either directly or indirectly, by the information contained in this book.

List of Abbreviations

BMI: Body mass index

CDC: Centers for Disease Control

DOB: Date of birth

HFZ: Healthy Fitness Zone

PE: physical education

INTRODUCTION

In 2007, I began college (hopefully for the last time), and in the course of a year, I had to take a multicultural education course. During the course, students were required to write a paper on discrimination, with specific topics approved by the professor before starting research. I told my professor I wanted to write about discrimination regarding obesity. She looked at me with a puzzled look on her face and asked me to explain, which I did. Her only response before approving my topic was that I make sure to show a connection to education, not just discrimination. The research I encountered was mind-boggling, unforgettable, and now I believe a spark to help others.

I found a research study (Puhl & Brownell, 2001), from the 1960s, in which a researcher set out to determine if children discriminated against their same-age, overweight peers. Children were given pictures of children with physical disabilities, such as facial disfigurements, and of an obese child. The children were instructed to rate the pictures in order of whom they would most want as their friend to whom they would least want as a friend. The researcher discovered that the majority of the children rated the obese child as the child they would least want as their friend. Documentation indicates this discrimination starts as early as age three, and it has been said the obese person is the last acceptable target of discrimination.

Forty years later, the overweight child continues to experience constant psychological beatings in social situations, more common for the overweight or obese student than not (Bailes, 2006). For these students, every social situation can cause them to prefer to be alone as opposed to socializing. This can lead to a vicious cycle of discontentment and depression, for some leading to suicide. The number one reason for peer rejection is being overweight, and overweight students are often rejected by their overweight peers (Renck Jalongo, 1999). These same students also experience pain and discrimination by those directly responsible for their care and well-being—their parents and teachers (Banks, 2006; Puhl & Brownell, 2001; Tiggeman & Anesbury, 2000).

In one study (Teachman & Brownell, 2001), overweight children as young as nine years old reported they had significantly lower self-esteem than their non-overweight peers. In addition, the overweight children believe the reason they are teased, have fewer friends, and are excluded from games and sports is due to their weight. In another study (Puhl & Brownell, 2001), researchers reported that students indicated the most common critics were their peers, and the most common place for such occurrences was at school. Students reported experiencing discrimination in high school, junior high school, middle school, and even in preschool. The research stated (Renck Jalongo, 1999), "Among all of the insults that children can hurl at one another, fat is the one that can hurt the most." Unfortunately, many students are becoming targets of cruelty, in places they have to go every day: home and school.

Regrettably, the discrimination is not stopping there. Today, discrimination is going on in colleges, college admissions, employment, doctors' offices, hospitals, healthcare facilities, airlines, jury selections, and even among relatives (NEA, 1999; Puhl & Brownell, 2001; Renck Jalongo, 1999; Teachman & Brownell, 2001; Tiggemann & Anesbury, 2000).

Lately it seems the news is flooded with stories, research studies, and statistical information regarding the dramatic increase in childhood obesity. The staggering statistics are affecting all ages, from infants to the elderly, races, socioeconomic levels, and countries around the world (Goel et al, 2004). Even more staggering are the results from a recent research study that includes nine-month-old babies and indicates a dramatic number of babies are already in the overweight to obese range before their first birthday (CDC, 2010; Ogden et al., 2010). Further, research states (Malecka-Tendera & Mazur, 2006; USDHHS, 2010) this early entrance into the overweight to obese range may be a predictor of a lifetime of obesity. If drastic changes are not put in place, childhood obesity can lead to a myriad of problems that can negatively affect a person's life at any age. Negative effects of childhood obesity include physical, medical, educational, and social/emotional areas.

In this book, we will get into the specifics of each of these areas. In addition, this book will cover the following topics:

- Overall statistics regarding childhood obesity

- Physical activity

- Physical fitness

- Data and research regarding childhood obesity

- How childhood obesity may affect you

- Developing a plan so you do not become a statistic; and

- A Healthy For Life lifestyle

It is my hope that this book will meet a few goals for you as you read. First, by reading this book, you will better understand the big picture of what childhood obesity is, including research, statistics, and how it may relate to you or someone you know. A second goal is that you will learn how *not* to be included in all the statistics I give, because I do not want you to experience all the negative effects we will discuss. A third goal is that you learn to live a life full of good health, free of ailments caused by obesity. A final goal is that you share the information and knowledge you gain by reading this book with others, maybe a friend or family member who may need the help; we can call it an extra reward for which we can all be thankful!

Before you continue reading, I must say one thing that I hope you keep in mind as you read this book, especially at times when you read something that may discourage you. I am writing this book to provide you with information regarding a disease: childhood obesity. It is not my intention to point the finger at the reader, even at times when statistics or stories may appear to be written specifically about you. When you read a story and know exactly what I am talking about, please do not think I mean to hurt your feelings or that I am being mean or ugly. Always remember, it is my sole intent to help you *not* be included in the negative statistics and stories I write about.

Chapter 1:
So What's the Big Deal—Overall Statistics Regarding Childhood Obesity

My first two goals of this book are that you will understand what childhood obesity is and learn how to keep from becoming one of those statistics. The title of this book is *It's NOT about Childhood Obesity; It Is about Being Healthy for Life*. If you do not want to be a part of something, you must first fully understand what that something is. Therefore, as we start chapter one, I will explain all of this right off the bat. When you finish reading the first chapter, you will ideally not only be knowledgeable about childhood obesity, but you truly will not want to be a part of the statistics. If you are already a part of the statistics, I hope this book gives you the knowledge to start your new journey of being healthy for life!

What is childhood obesity? Obesity is defined by the Centers for Disease Control and Prevention (CDC, 2010) as two weight-status categories above a healthy weight category and includes a percentile range of eighty-fifth to ninety-fifth percentile. There are four weight-status categories, which include the following:

Body Mass Index Weight Status Category – Percentile Range

Weight Status Category	Percentile Range
Underweight	Less than the 5th percentile
Healthy weight	5th percentile to less than the 85th percentile
Overweight	85th to less than the 95th percentile
Obese	Equal to or greater than the 95th percentile

Source: CDC

Which weight-status category a child or teen is in is determined by a Body Mass Index, or BMI. A BMI can be calculated for children and teens ages two through nineteen, and of course for adults. BMI is an inexpensive, easy-to-perform, and reliable indicator of how much body fat a person is carrying on his or her body. To calculate your BMI, you will need the following information:

- date of birth;
- date of measurement (the date height and weight were taken);
- sex;
- height to nearest eighth inch; and
- weight to nearest quarter pound

In the Notes section, I have listed this information, and I have left room for you to write your numbers next to each question. When you get time, go to the website listed in the Notes section and enter your information, and it will calculate your BMI for you. For children and teens, BMI is specific according to age and gender; however, for adults, BMI is not specific according to age and gender, but rather merely based on height and weight. The specific formula for adults to calculate BMI is as follows: Weight (in pounds) / Height (in inches)^2 x 703.

While we are talking about weight categories and BMI, let's look at some real people and what their BMI is and the information obtained from the website. I grabbed a few of my nieces and a nephew, and we are going to look at their information, including date of birth, date of measurement, sex, height, and weight. Then we will get results that will include a BMI, percentile, and weight-status category. The website will also provide some suggestions on what the information means and what should be done, which is helpful.

	GWYNN	MATTHEW	EMILY
Height	5' 1"	5' 8"	5' 5"
Weight	105	140	127
Date Measured	4/4/2012	4/4/2012	4/4/2012
DOB	5/21/1998	11/13/1996	8/8/1994
Gender	F	M	F
BMI	19.8	21.3	21.1
Percentile Range	57th	65th	49th
Weight Status Category	Healthy	Healthy	Healthy

Source: Vaca Durr, 2012

As you can tell, all three are in their teenage years; the girls are fourteen and seventeen, and Matthew is fifteen. Gwynn, a female, is five feet one inch and weighs 105 pounds. Matthew is a male who is five feet eight inches and weighs 140 pounds. In addition, Emily is a five-foot-five-inch female weighing 127 pounds. All three are in a healthy weight-status category; however, the website still provides information for participants. For example, for Gwynn the website states, "Regardless of the current BMI—for—age category, help your child or teen develop healthy weight habits and keep track on BMI—for—age." Additionally, the website warns that Gwynn should 1) eat healthily; 2) participate in physical activity, preferably every day of the week; and 3) limit television viewing.

Since many younger children are experiencing childhood obesity, I wanted to look at the heights, weights, and BMIs of some younger children as well. The following information is on a five-year-old boy and a six-year-old girl, both about to enter first grade, who are not in a healthy weight-status category. However, both children could be in a healthy weight-status category by losing less than ten pounds. The boy could lose eight pounds and go from an obese weight-status category to a healthy weight-status category; a mere two pounds would put the girl in a healthy weight-status category.

Name:	Chase	Savannah
Birth Date:	9/14/2006	10/27/2005
Date of Measurement:	3/27/2012	3/27/2012
Sex:	M	F
Height, to nearest 1/8 inch:	46"	48"
Weight, to nearest ¼ pound:	58 lbs.	58 lbs.
BMI	19.3	17.7
Percentile	96	88
Weight-Status Category	obese	overweight

These two children are not quite a year apart, and Savannah is two inches taller than Chase. However, both children will be entering first grade, and they both weigh fifty-eight pounds. Chase is in the obese weight-status category, and the information provided by the CDC warns that he needs to be seen by a healthcare provider for further assessment. Savannah is listed as overweight, and the information provided by the CDC warns that although not obese, she has the potential for becoming obese, and prevention is important. For Chase's current height, forty-six inches or three feet ten inches, he needs to weigh fifty pounds, eight pounds less than his current weight, to be in a healthy weight category. For Savannah's current height, forty-eight inches or four feet, she needs to weigh fifty-six pounds, two pounds less, to be in a healthy weight category. Keep in mind, your BMI changes as you get taller, get older, and of course, as your weight changes, even by five pounds. So *never think that just because you are in one weight-status category today, you will* stay *in that weight-status category forever.*

Now that we know what obesity and BMI mean, let's look at some statistics and research so we can learn more about this subject. After all, if we do not want to be included in the childhood obesity statistics, we need to know more about them. In an effort to define this epidemic of obesity, which is widespread throughout the world, researchers (Goel et al., 2004) have used the term "globesity." Globesity is defined as the global epidemic of obesity or how obesity is affecting so many countries throughout the world. I am going to give you a lot of statistics, age ranges, and numbers, but I promise I will explain all of them, so you fully understand what they mean.

In May 2010, the White House Task Force on Childhood Obesity wrote a report to the president titled "Solving the Problem of Childhood Obesity within a Generation." The challenge listed in the report was that the childhood obesity epidemic in America is a national health crisis. *In 2007–2008, according to the report, 31.7 percent of children ages two to nineteen are either overweight or already obese, roughly thirty-two out of one hundred.* So what does that mean? It means that one out of every three children aged two to nineteen is in the overweight or obese weight-status category. The report also stated that the negative effects of obesity cause 112,000 deaths every year in the United States.

On top of that (White House Task Force on Childhood Obesity, 2010), one-third of all children born in the year 2000 and after are expected to develop diabetes. We will talk more about diabetes in chapter 5. Diabetes is a negative effect of being overweight or obese, and statistics show if you were born in 2000, you have a one in three chance of becoming a diabetic. It is also estimated that the costs of being overweight or obese during childhood total $3 billion per year in direct medical costs (White House Task Force on Childhood Obesity, 2010). This is an enormous amount of money spent just on medical costs as a result of being overweight or obese. Just think what could be done with an extra $3 billion. It could be spent on science labs or better electronic equipment for schools.

Let's look at a few more statistics regarding globesity. This childhood obesity epidemic did not just begin in 2000. According to data from the CDC (2010), from 1964 to 1970, roughly 4.6 percent of children aged twelve to nineteen were in the overweight category. At that time, children aged twelve to nineteen in the obese category were not even mentioned, probably because there were so few. This statistic means about five children aged twelve to nineteen out of one hundred were at a weight calculated in the overweight category. Research also shows that during the 1960s (CDC, 2010), 4 percent of children aged six to eleven were considered in the overweight

weight-status category, roughly four out of one hundred. These numbers are much smaller than the 31.7 percent of children in 2007–2008 who were calculated in the overweight to obese range.

By 1999–2000 (CDC, 2010), these numbers exploded, increasing threefold, with 15.5 percent of children aged twelve to nineteen considered to be in the overweight range, previously only 4.6 percent. So out of those one hundred children, now about sixteen were calculated to be in the overweight category. In 2001 (Small, Anderson, & Mazurek Melnyk, 2007), data was also revealed on a second age group, including the weight-status category of overweight children and obese children. *By 2001, it was estimated that 21 percent of children aged two to five had a BMI that put them in the overweight or obese weight-status category.* Children aged two to five are not even in first grade yet. Unfortunately, the statistics get worse. *In 2007–2008 (Ogden et al., 2010), calculations began for children even younger; researchers discovered that 9.5 percent of infants and toddlers were already at or above the ninety-fifth percentile according to weight and length. The ninety-fifth percentile is in the obese weight-status category,* and unfortunately, this percentage does not include the overweight infants and toddlers from birth to age two.

Although the obesity rates are not as high in some states throughout the United States—for example, Oregon (Trust for America's Health, 2007)—other countries are also experiencing the national epidemic of childhood obesity that the United States is experiencing, countries such as the United Kingdom, New Zealand, Finland, and Brazil (Taras & Potts-Datema, 2005). In addition, Thailand, Mexico, and Japan are experiencing high numbers of obese children. Worldwide (Malecka-Tendera & Mazur, 2006), there are more than a billion people who weigh in at the obese range, that weight equal to or greater than the ninety-fifth percentile according to BMI. Additionally, worldwide, 22 million children age five or under weigh in as either overweight or obese (Malecka-Tendera & Mazur, 2006). Results of the first National Health Examination Survey (Pyle et al., 2006) in the early 1960s indicated that four percent of children aged six to eleven and five percent of twelve- to nineteen–year-olds were categorized as overweight. Furthermore, the data stated that the incidence of overweight and obesity is more common among minority females and the lower socioeconomic status population. As you can distinguish by these numbers, the rates have made enormous growth.

You may wonder why childhood obesity is such a big issue in children. *The reason childhood obesity is such a big issue is because today in America, the most common health problem in young people is being overweight* (Ganz, 2003). Childhood is the most influential time for a person to establish physical activity behaviors that they can carry with them throughout their life and can make positive changes on into adulthood (Prosser & Jiang, 2008).

Obesity is often the result of an imbalance between caloric intake and physical inactivity (APHA, 2012). A continued imbalance eventually leads to becoming overweight or obese. However, the good news is that imbalance can be balanced out. Research shows (Malecka-Tendera & Mazur, 2006) that children who are not physically active and then become overweight or obese as children will most likely become adults who are not physically active and therefore continue being overweight or obese into adulthood. If during childhood you do not learn to lead an active life, how can you become an adult who will live an active life? It is similar to learning to ride a bike. If you don't learn to ride a bike as a child, chances are slim you will learn to ride a bike as an adult. Nevertheless, that does not mean you can never learn to ride a bike *or* be a physically active adult.

By now, I hope you fully understand what the big issue is regarding childhood obesity. We have talked about the definition of overweight and obese, the different weight-status categories, and what a BMI or body mass index is. We also calculated a few people's BMI and saw how five pounds can make a difference and that once you are in one weight-status category, it does not mean you will stay there. I also listed a website so you can find out exactly what your BMI is. Additionally, we looked at statistics and data from the 1960s to 2008 of children at different ages and weight-status categories and the changes that occurred throughout the years. I hope you think about all you have learned and go to the website to calculate your own BMI. Use your current BMI as a baseline to get into a healthy weight-status category. You might be like Savannah, and a few pounds will get you into a healthier weight-status category by increasing your physical activity, eating healthier foods, and limiting your television time. Just knowing what your BMI is will help you. Keep in mind what I said before: if you are in the overweight or obese weight-status category, under no circumstances do you have to stay there. However, it is up to you to get out of a particular weight-status category if you are overweight or obese. In the next few chapters, we will talk about ways to get out of an overweight or obese weight-status category and start your healthy-for-life lifestyle.

Chapter 1 Notes

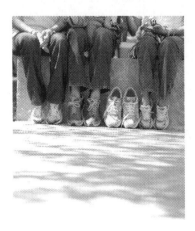

Source: jcannonphotography

DEFINITIONS

GLOBESITY: The global epidemic of obesity or how obesity is affecting so many countries throughout the globe (Ganz, 2003).

ADDITIONAL INFORMATION

TofindyourspecificBMI,accordingtoyourheight,weight, age, and gender; you can go to the following website at the Centers for Disease Control (CDC) and Prevention: *http://apps.nccd.cdc.gov/dnpabmi/*

Formula for Adults to Calculate a BMI:

Weight (in pounds) / Height (in inches)^2 x 703

A Recap of Years, Percentiles, Age Ranges, and Weight-Status Categories:

Year	%	Ages	Weight-status category
1963–1970	4.6	12–19	Overweight
1999–2000	15.5	12–19	Overweight
2001	21.0	2–5	Overweight or obese
2007–2008	9.5	Infants-toddlers	Obese
2007–2008	31.7	2–19	Overweight or obese

Of course, there are additional statistics that could close the gap between 1963–1970 and 2007–2008, but I wanted to show the difference over a span of years and what it has become today.

TO DO

Information You Need to Calculate Your BMI:

- Birth Date: _____

- Date of Measurement: _____

- Sex: _____

- Height, to nearest 1/8 inch:_____

- Weight, to nearest ¼ pound:_____

KEY POINT

The reason childhood obesity is such a big issue is because today in America, the most common health problem in young people is being overweight.

Chapter 2: Physical Activity, Why Is it So Important?

The Centers for Disease Control (CDC, 2010) published a state indicator report on physical activity in 2010, stating that physical activity is essential to overall health. In addition, it listed four benefits of physical activity, stating that physical activity can help control weight, reduce the risk of heart disease and some cancers, strengthen bones and muscles, and improve mental health. For young children, physical activity has additional benefits. Physical activity also helps improve fine and gross motor skills, coordination, balance and control, hand-eye coordination, and strength, dexterity, and flexibility.

So what is physical activity? Essentially, physical activity is getting up and moving around or getting active. For children, being physically active could include playing a game of chase, riding a scooter, playing on a jungle gym, or running up a hill so you can slide down on a saucer. For older children and teens, being physically active could include taking the dog for a walk, going swimming, riding a bicycle or scooter, going out on rollerblades, participating in a sport, or going for a walk or run.

The United States Department of Health and Human Services and the Centers for Disease Control (2008) recommend that children and teens get a minimum of *sixty minutes of physical activity every single day.*

Physical activity encompasses bodily motion resulting in energy expenditure that is produced by skeletal muscles (Schumacher & Queen, 2007). Physical activity is closely related to exercise, but if you think about it, people typically consider adults to be exercising when they are going for a run or out for a walk and consider children to be *playing* when they are participating in the same activity. So is age the only difference between physical activity and exercise? Actually, the difference between physical activity and exercise is that exercise is defined as being planned, structured, and repetitive, whereas physical activity is performed to improve or maintain physical fitness (Schumacher & Queen, 2007). Be aware that physical activity, exercise, and physical fitness (a topic we will discuss in the next chapter) are not one and the same; however, they are all closely related. Although not being physically fit will not make you overweight, not being physically active or engaging in regular physical activity will lead you on the path to becoming overweight and obese (Spiegel & Foulk, 2006). So, whenever you can, try to add some physical activity into your daily schedule. An easy way to do so is to try to make physical activity fun; it increases the chances you will continue.

The United States Department of Health and Human Services (2008) classifies physical activity into four categories. Each of the categories includes the number of minutes per week, the intensity of the physical activity, and the overall health benefit at that level. The low-level category includes less than 150 minutes of physical activity per week, at a low intensity, but still has some overall health benefits. This level would include twenty minutes or less of low-intensity physical activity daily. However, there are still some health benefits, even at these low levels. Even if you have a medical issue that does not allow you to be physically active 60 minutes per day, try for 150 minutes per week (less than 20 minutes per day), at least at a low level. Even with this low level of physical activity, at least it is better than not being physically active at all.

The chart below shows which overall health benefits are associated with each level of physical activity. At the medium level of physical activity, a person engages in roughly twenty to forty minutes of physical activity per day, providing substantial overall health benefits. The highest level of physical activity includes forty-three or more minutes of physical activity per day, which provides additional health benefits, although the extent of those health benefits is not specific.

Classification of Total Weekly Amounts of Aerobic Physical Activity into Four Categories

Levels of Physical Activity	Range of Moderate-Intensity Minutes a Week	Summary of Overall Health Benefits	Comment
Inactive	No activity beyond baseline	None	Being inactive is unhealthy.
Low	Activity beyond baseline but fewer than 150 minutes a week	Some	Low levels of activity are clearly preferable to an inactive lifestyle
Medium	150 minutes to 300 minutes a week	Substantial	Activity at the high end of this range has additional and more extensive health benefits than activity at the low end.
High	More than 300 minutes a week	Additional	Current science does not allow researchers to identify an upper limit of activity above which there are no additional health benefits.

Source: USDHHS

What other benefits does physical activity have? According to researchers (Cook, 2005), by engaging in physical activity, new brain cells begin to grow. Some researchers equate physical activity to "Miracle-Gro" for the brain. You may recall "Miracle-Gro" is put on plants to make them grow and look fabulous! Now doesn't that make you want to engage in physical activity, just knowing what it can do for your brain? Other researchers (Taras, 2005; Vail, 2006) equate physical activity to a brain workout, causing the body to improve general circulation, increase blood flow to the brain, and increase the levels of norepinephrine and endorphins. Increased levels of norepinephrine and endorphins allow you to reduce stress, improve your mood, and be calm. Going on a walk with family can be a good idea for everyone to improve their mood, calm down, and reduce stress.

But there are other benefits to physical activity (Taras, 2005). It enhances synaptic activity in the brain, increasing communication among brain cells. Physical activity helps brain function, improves academic performance, and decreases health problems. Students who engage in physical activity experience lower incidence of depression and engage in fewer risky behaviors (CDE, 2002; NASPE, 2002; SSDHPER, 2005; Spiegel & Foulk, 2006; Trost, 2007; Trost & van der Mars, 2010; USDHHS, 2008; USHR, 2008). Even with all these benefits of physical activity, research shows 50 percent of Americans aged twelve to twenty-one are inactive (Pyle et al., 2006; Spiegel & Foulk, 2006; USDHHS, 1999). This means one out of two children aged twelve to twenty-one does not participate in physical activity, nor do they receive all the benefits gained. Another researcher (Trachtenberg, 2007) stated that 34 percent of youth aged twelve to nineteen would flunk an eight-minute treadmill test. If ten students, aged twelve to nineteen, were given a test and had to walk on a treadmill for eight minutes, a third of them would not be able to successfully complete the eight-minute walk. The students were not told they had to run or even go at a fast pace; they just had to walk for eight minutes. Only seven of the ten students were successful.

What kinds of physical activity should you engage in? According to the United States Department of Health and Human Services, children and adolescents should participate in the following types and amounts of physical activity:

Physical Activity Guidelines for Children and Adolescents

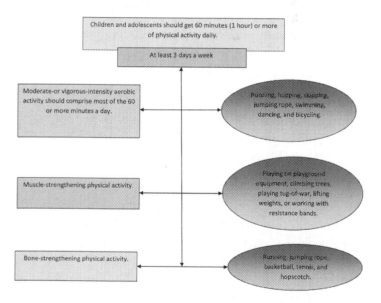

Children and adolescents should get 60 minutes (1 hour) or more of physical activity daily.

At least 3 days a week

Moderate-or vigorous-intensity aerobic activity should comprise most of the 60 or more minutes a day.

Running, hopping, skipping, jumping rope, swimming, dancing, and bicycling.

Muscle-strengthening physical activity.

Playing on playground equipment, climbing trees, playing tug-of-war, lifting weights, or working with resistance bands.

Bone-strengthening physical activity.

Running, jumping rope, basketball, tennis, and hopscotch.

Source: USDHHS

As you can tell from the chart, the United States Department of Health and Human Services recommends sixty minutes of physical activity daily and at least three days a week in the following categories: moderate- or vigorous-intensity aerobic activity, muscle-strengthening physical activity, and bone-strengthening physical activity. If you are unsure what activities you could do for each category, here are some examples:

> For moderate- or vigorous-intensity aerobic activity, you could go for a run, hop, skip, jump rope, swim, dance, or ride a bicycle.

> For muscle-strengthening activities you could play on playground equipment, climbing trees, playing tug-of-war, and activities such as lifting weights or working with resistance bands.

> For bone-strengthening, you could do some activities that were also listed in the moderate- or vigorous-intensity aerobic activity area, such as running and jumping rope, or you could also play basketball or tennis or a game of hopscotch.

I hope in each area there was at least one activity listed that you enjoy or that you know of activities similar to the ones listed that you enjoy!

Due to budget cuts, many school districts are experiencing cuts in the area of physical education. In 2006 (Trost, 2007), fewer than 10 percent of school districts across the United States were offering daily physical education. The following chart shows the percentage of schools in 2006 that provided physical education on a daily basis. Considering current national budget cuts, those numbers could be even lower within the next few years. With obesity rates as high as they are, some districts need to reconsider cutting physical activity out of the schedule.

Percentage of Schools Providing Daily PE in 2006	Percentage
Elementary Schools	3.8%
Middle Schools	7.9%
High Schools	2.1%

Source: Trost, 2007

Considering the high percentages of childhood obesity and low percentages of schools offering daily physical education, it is of utmost importance for children and teens to make sure they are including physical activity in their schedule every day. Sadly, many children and teens are surrounded by role models who do not participate in physical activity or exercise (Schumacher & Queen, 2007), role models such as parents, teachers, school and church leaders, coaches, aunts and uncles, and grandparents. For this reason, it is critical for you to know how important physical activity is in your life and to be a person that adds physical activity to your life every day in an effort to be healthy for life!

In this chapter, we have learned:

- What physical activity means

- How much physical activity we should participate in daily

- What types of physical activity need to be included

- The benefits and importance of physical activity and what it does for you

We need to try to be a good role model when it comes to adding physical activity to our daily lives because many of our role models are not. Being a good role model could help them become a better role model too.

This information is important because we do not want to become one of the statistics we have been reading about. We want to live healthy for life. You may have a friend or family member who needs help or who is battling childhood obesity, or even adult obesity. What you are learning will be a benefit not just today but for the remainder of your life and can be a tool to help others. In our next chapter, we will discuss physical fitness.

Chapter 2 Notes

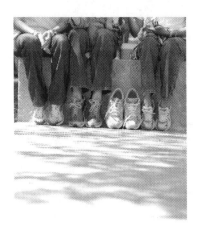

Source: jcannonphotography

DEFINITIONS

> PHYSICAL ACTIVITY: Bodily motion resulting in energy expenditure that is produced by skeletal muscles and is performed to improve or maintain physical fitness (Schumacher & Queen, 2007).

> EXERCISE: Activity that is planned, structured, and repetitive (Schumacher & Queen, 2007).

TO DO

How much physical activity do you get per day? ____

_____

_____

Do you think you should get more physical activity? Yes or No

Try to make sure when you participate in physical activity that you are having fun!

Could you pass an eight-minute treadmill test? Try it! Go for a walk and time yourself! It doesn't have to be on a treadmill; just walk eight minutes! Could you do it?

Please say you can ... I'm cheering for you!

List ways you can get your friends and family members (who you know need more physical activity) to get out and get active?

_____

_____

_____

_____

_____

_____

KEY POINT

Keep in mind the CDC recommends sixty minutes per day.

EVERY DAY!

Or at least days that end in "y."

Chapter 3: Physical Fitness

Physical fitness is a subset of both physical activity and exercise, but keep in mind, just because you are physically active or participate in exercise does not mean that you are automatically physically fit (Schumacher & Queen, 2007). It is worth noting, the only way to increase your physical fitness is to engage in physical activity or exercise *on a regular basis.* Sounds like a big circle, doesn't it?

The lack of physical fitness levels in children has led to the current obesity levels referred to earlier as "globesity." As previously stated, childhood obesity or obesity during adolescence leads to adult obesity if positive measures are not taken to correct the imbalance. Research shows (Pyle et al., 2006; Spiegel & Foulk, 2006; TEA, 2008; USDHHS, 1999; USHR, 2008) that as children get older, their level of physical activity decreases. Why do you think that as you get older, your level of physical activity goes down? Let's think about that. Who do you think is more physically fit, a third grader or a fifth grader? Probably the third grader, right? In third grade, it is cool to run around the playground, hang upside down on the monkey bars, or just run back and forth aimlessly for hours.

In fifth grade, the books get heavier, the homework increases, and the level of coolness decreases regarding running aimlessly back and forth or hanging upside down on the monkey bars. Now let's look at two other groups of students. Do you think the elementary student is more physically fit or the high school student? I hope you said the elementary student. I have many nephews and nieces and was a schoolteacher in both elementary and secondary, and I promise, the older students get, the less they want to hang upside down on monkey bars or play tag or ride a Big Wheel.

There are a number of additional reasons why physical fitness levels decrease with each passing birthday. A recent study conducted throughout the State of Texas (TEA, 2008) shows just how much our physical fitness levels decrease with each passing birthday.

In 2007, Texas was ranked as the seventh-fattest state in the nation, having the seventh-largest number of obese children aged ten to seventeen, with 19.1 percent considered obese. As a result, Texas passed Senate Bill 530 requiring all students throughout the state, in grades three to twelve, to be tested in the area of physical fitness. As a result, there were approximately 2.6 million students tested during the 2007–2008 school year. A supporter of the bill stated, "In education, there are fundamentals and there are electives. Good health is as fundamental as reading, writing, and arithmetic, a lesson students *must* learn."

To test students' physical fitness, the state used a test called the Fitnessgram. The Fitnessgram (Human Kinetics, 2008) was developed in 1982 by Dr. Kenneth Cooper and the Cooper Institute in Dallas Texas along with a team of advisors, all recognized as experts in the field of pediatric exercise science.

The Fitnessgram includes three areas of testing, based on age and gender. The three areas include:

- aerobic capacity

- body composition

- muscular strength, endurance, and flexibility

In addition, there is a list of testing options for each area of testing. The complete list can be found in the chapter 3 notes section.

On the Fitnessgram, to test aerobic capacity, a student will take a PACER test. PACER is an acronym for Progressive Aerobic Cardiovascular Endurance Run, and the objective is to run as long as possible across a twenty-meter space at a specific pace. Aerobic capacity can also be tested on a one-mile run or walk.

The second assessment area is body composition, which is assessed according to your BMI or a skin-fold test, which is another way to assess body-fat percentage. We talked about BMI in chapter 1, where we also listed the formula and I hope you calculated your BMI. A third way to assess body composition is from a bioelectric impedance analysis device. To pass this area or be in the healthy fitness zone, a student's BMI has to be between a certain range of numbers according to their age and gender.

The third assessment area—muscular strength, endurance, and flexibility—is assessed with four different tests. The first is a curl-up test, and the objective is to complete as many curl-ups as possible. The second is a trunk-lift test, and the objective is to lift the upper body off the floor using the muscles in your back and hold the position while it is measured. The next test is the push-up test, and the objective is to complete as many push-ups as possible in a given amount of time. The final test is a sit-and-reach test, which tests flexibility; the objective is to be able to reach a specified distance on both the right and left sides of your body.

All tests are specific to the Fitnessgram, but it gives you an idea of how physical fitness is tested and what you need to do in a physical fitness test. You can go to *www.cooperinstitute.org* to learn more about the Fitnessgram, health and fitness resources, the youth zone, and much more. In addition, your physical education teacher may be able to give you more information. The Fitnessgram and the President's Challenge are the two most widely used physical fitness assessment instruments in the United States.

I mention the Fitnessgram, the three areas of testing, and the specific tests under each area to provide you with the information on how physical fitness is tested. Aerobic capacity and body composition include one area that has a few options on testing. However, the third area tested, muscular strength, endurance, and flexibility, includes more tests and focuses on more areas of the body.

So what are muscular strength, endurance, and flexibility? This area of testing focuses on how strong you are, how long you can last, and how flexible you are. Babies are typically very flexible. Have you ever seen a baby put his feet or toes in his mouth? Now that takes flexibility. But that same baby is not very strong and cannot last very long before he is taking a snooze. As the baby gets older, he typically gets stronger and is able to last longer if allowed opportunities to play and explore or engage in physical activity. As you can imagine, after a baby gets stronger (strength) and is able to last longer (endurance), if the little child does not continue to engage in physical activity as he gets older, the strength and endurance disappear, as does the flexibility. I mean, can you still put your toes in your mouth?

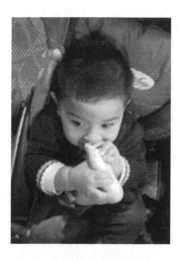

**Just to see if you can (or not).
So how is your flexibility since you
were eighteen months old?**

Being overweight can also diminish or decrease a child's muscular strength, endurance, and flexibility. I have seen overweight children, aged four to six, in classes like martial arts and gymnastics, who cannot roll over and tumble or kick their leg up, and children at soccer camp who cannot last forty-five minutes without having to stop and rest repeatedly, even with numerous water breaks. By knowing what you now know about physical-fitness testing, you can see how the overweight child may not be as strong, if they have to lift their own weight, such as in sit-ups, or participate in physical activities for an extended period. Additionally, it is easy to see how the weight will hinder flexibility. It is my intent that by discussing a physical fitness test, you will better understand what is involved, what is tested, and can better understand our next section, which explains the results of the first year of testing physical fitness in Texas that started during the 2007–2008 school year. I share these results to show you how quick fitness can decrease and at an early age if not included as a daily part of your life. Therefore, it is important that you maintain physical activity and fitness throughout your life to ensure you stay healthy for life.

Earlier in this chapter, we talked about how as youth get older, their level of physical activity decreases, and they can no longer put their toes in their mouth. The first year of physical-fitness testing began in Texas during the 2007–2008 school year, using the Fitnessgram. The following chart not only shows the percentage of students by grade level testing out in the Healthy Fitness Zone but also shows how the more birthdays you have decreases physical ability. However, first you need to know what a Healthy Fitness Zone or HFZ is.

The Fitnessgram is a criterion-referenced test, based on levels of fitness needed for good health, set specifically for boys and girls of various ages. It is not based on class averages or peer comparisons. Testing in the Healthy Fitness Zone is like passing a test. The Healthy Fitness Zone is the standard needed in each test, according to gender and age, and determines if you pass a test or not. Therefore, if according to your age and gender, you score the appropriate number needed on one of the tests, you are considered in a Healthy Fitness Zone, or in other words, you passed the test. If you do not score the appropriate number needed on a specific test, you are not in a Healthy Fitness Zone on that test, according to your age and gender. Since there are five tests and a body composition, you can score in the Healthy Fitness Zone up to six times or as low as zero.

The chart below actually fits in both this chapter on physical fitness and the next chapter, in which we talk about data and research, so keep this page handy. In the next chapter, we will reference it again with additional data on this research study.

2007 - 2008 Data FITNESSGRAM® Data
(% Achieving Healthy Fitness Zone on all 6 tests)

Grade	Total # Tested	Girls (%)	Boys (%)
3	102,342	33.25	28.6
4	80,539	28.5	21.14
5	66,798	23.82	17.89
6	60,663	23.08	17.6
7	55,441	21.32	17.26
8	48,971	18.99	17.88
9	39,456	13.9	15.04
10	28,650	12.42	13.7
11	21,152	10.68	12.24
12	13,040	8.18	8.96

Students Assessed: 2,658,665
Districts Submitting: 1,074 (84.77%)

Source: TEA, 2008

The first column is the grade level of the students tested and includes grades three to twelve. The second column is the total number of students tested across the State of Texas, according to that grade level (in the first column). The third and fourth columns break up the total percentage of students by gender who tested in the Healthy Fitness Zone or passed all six of the tests.

In third grade, out of the 102,342 total students tested, 33.25 percent of the girls and 28.60 percent of the boys tested in the Healthy Fitness Zone. As you look down the columns, or in the higher grades, you will notice the percentages decreasing at each passing grade level. Alternatively, as the grade level increases, the percentage of students passing all six tests on the Fitnessgram decreases. *This chart shows you that at higher grade levels, the percentage of students passing all six tests on the Fitnessgram decreases.* Actually, the chart shows you a few more things.

The chart shows that a higher percentage of girls successfully passed all six tests than boys in third grade and on through eighth grade. Then, the chart shows at ninth grade, a higher percentage of boys successfully passed all six tests on the Fitnessgram, whereas 1.14 percent fewer girls than boys scored in the Healthy Fitness Zone. The chart also shows that in third grade, roughly 33 percent of girls and 28 percent of boys tested at physically fit, according to the Fitnessgram; but by twelfth grade, only 8.9 percent of boys and 8.1 percent of girls tested as physically fit. You may be thinking this was one state and one year, but the results in this research study follow current national research (Pyle et al., 2006; Spiegel & Foulk, 2006; USDHHS, 1999) that state *as children get older, their level of physical fitness decreases*, therefore, it is up to you to make sure this does not happen to you.

During the second year of testing in Texas, in 2008–2009, the results had similar findings, which we will discuss in the next chapter. But a word of caution: girls are getting more and more fit; guys, you better watch out!

The Fitnessgram assesses students in the areas of aerobic capacity, body composition, and muscular strength, endurance, and flexibility. Each assessment is age- and gender-specific, which means an eight-year-old girl in third grade does not have to make the same score as a ten-year-old boy in fifth grade to be successful.

In this and the previous chapter, we have discussed physical activity and physical fitness. If you are not physically active or think you need to be more physically active in order to pass a physical fitness test, then now may be a good time to get started. A great way to get started is by collecting data; you can see where you are today, as well as the progress you make in the coming weeks and months, maybe even years. So, go walk a mile and set a timer to see how long it takes. Keep walking and try to walk a mile at least three times per week. Then, in two weeks, see if your one-mile time has decreased. The more you walk that one mile, the easier it will be.

If one mile is easy, start with two or three miles, maybe five. For more active people, those who exercise regularly and are past one mile, run instead of walk a few miles and keep track of the length of time it takes over time, to determine if your time decreases. By knowing how long it takes you to complete a mile or even three (if that is where you started), it will help you in a month or two to know if you are cutting your time. Continue to keep track; this will show your progress, and if you are like me, it will keep you excited and motivated to do better.

In the appendices, I put a copy of my current exercise chart. I started using this after I got serious about walking/running on a regular basis, which took a few years. I also add an S for swimming, B for biking, H for hills, A for abs, etc. At the bottom of the chart, I calculate those times or miles in addition to the miles of walking/running. You should do whatever is easy for you. Modify the chart so it is a useful tool to help you become successful in participating in physical activity on a regular basis.

In this chapter, we talked about physical fitness and its importance. We talked about how being physically active and exercising will help you be physically fit. Then we talked about what caused the entire State of Texas to begin testing the physical fitness of all students in grades three to twelve, using the Fitnessgram. We learned how many researchers observe that, as children get older, their level of physical fitness decreases and saw those results in the Texas data. Now we are going to look at a little more data and research on childhood obesity and a little more on the testing in Texas.

Chapter 3 Notes

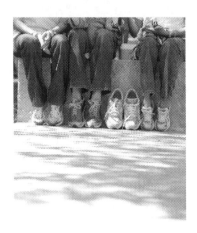

Source: jcannonphotography

DEFINITIONS

> PEDIATRIC EXERCISE SCIENCE: The study of exercise during childhood.

ADDITIONAL INFORMATION

A few reasons why our level of physical activity decreases with each passing birthday:

- You don't have recess anymore

- You grow too mature for Big Wheels, scooters, and stick horses

- As a teenager, who is there to play tag with anyway

- Why would you act like a superhero when you can just go to the movie?

- It is no longer "cool" to play chase games, hang upside down on the monkey bars, or run around all over being silly until you are finally tired enough to go to sleep.

Information on the Fitnessgram

The focus of Fitnessgram is on health-related fitness, as opposed to just sports performance. The long-term goal is by focusing on physical activity during childhood, children will grow up to be physically active adults who therefore are also healthy adults. An expert on the advisory team developed an acronym that expresses the philosophy of Fitnessgram. The acronym is H.E.L.P. and stands for *Health is available for Everyone for a Lifetime and it is Personal.* The acronym also serves as a reminder that improving the fitness of youth requires the H.E.L.P. of all, including parents, teachers, schools, family members, and the community, as well as yourself. Also, each letter of the acronym includes the following importance:

H: health comes from regular physical activity and the development of health-related fitness;

E: physical activity and fitness is for everyone, regardless of age, gender, or ability;

L: physical activity and fitness are for a lifetime; and

P: programs that concentrate on physical activity and fitness should be designed to meet personal needs and interests.

Fitnessgram tests according to area of testing and testing options for each area:

1. Aerobic Capacity

    - One-mile run/walk

    - PACER test stands for Progressive Aerobic Cardiovascular Endurance Run. The objective is to run as long as possible across a twenty-meter space at a specific pace.

    - Walk test, only validated to date on children thirteen years and older.

2. Body Composition

    - Percent body fat from skinfold measurements

    - Percent body fat from bioelectric impedance analysis (BIA) device

    - Body mass index from height and weight measurements

3. Muscular Strength, Endurance, and Flexibility

    - Abdominal strength and endurance:

        ○ Curl-up: the objective is to complete as many as possible to a cadence with a maximum of seventy-five.

    - Trunk extensor strength and endurance:

o   Trunk lift: the objective is to lift the upper body off the floor using the muscles of the back and hold the position to allow for the measurement.

- Upper body strength and endurance: the objective is to complete as many as possible at a rhythmic pace:

    o   Ninety-degree push-up

    o   Modified pull-up

    o   Flexed arm hang

- Flexibility: the objective is to be able to reach the specified distance on the right and left sides of the body:

    o   Back-saver sit and reach

    o   Shoulder stretch

Chapter 4: Childhood Obesity Data and Research

This chapter will be full of data and research from different studies on childhood obesity. Keep in mind what we talked about at the beginning of the book: I am writing this book to provide you with information regarding a disease or epidemic also termed globesity. I am *not* pointing a finger, although the data or research may hit home and sound like I am specifically talking about you. I am giving you data and research so as you get older, you will not be included in this type of research. However, if you are already in the group included in this research, I hope by reading this book you are provided the tools and information to change things for the positive, getting out of your current situation and any negatives included with your current situation, such as health problems you might be experiencing.

The data and research we will talk about in this chapter will be broken down into the following groups:

- 4.1 Being or Not Being Physically Active

- 4.2 How Being Physically Fit Can Help You in School

- 4.3 How People around You Affect You

We will talk about the research and offer a thorough explanation. The data and research we talk about in this chapter will also lead into the next chapter, where we talk about how obesity affects you, either as a child, a teen, or an adult. In addition, it is my intent that by knowing the facts, you will work hard not to experience obesity in your life, and you can even help those around you, like parents, siblings, or your best friend. You may even help save their life.

4.1 Being or Not Being Physically Active

According to the CDC (2008), children and adolescents should engage in sixty minutes or more of physical activity on a daily basis in three areas: aerobic, muscle-strengthening, and bone-strengthening. Additionally, the CDC stresses in the guidelines that it is important for young people to participate in physical activities that are not only age-appropriate and enjoyable but that also add variety to physical activity routines. The CDC guidelines include the following information in each area:

> Aerobic: most of the sixty or more minutes a day should be either moderate- or vigorous-intensity aerobic physical activity and should include vigorous-intensity physical activity at least three days a week.

> Muscle–strengthening: as part of their sixty or more minutes of daily physical activity, children and adolescents should include muscle-strengthening physical activity at least three days of the week.

Bone-strengthening: as part of their sixty or more minutes of daily physical activity, children and adolescents should include bone-strengthening physical activity at least three days of the week.

Did you notice some similarities? The three areas of physical activity you should engage in daily include aerobic, muscle-strengthening, and bone-strengthening; whereas the three areas of physical-fitness testing in the Fitnessgram include aerobic capacity, body composition, and muscular strength, endurance, and flexibility. The three areas are not exactly the same but do have many similarities.

So why is engaging in physical activity such a big deal? The following is a list of the benefits of engaging in physical activity (CDE, 2002; Cook, 2005; NASPE, 2002; SSDHPER, 2005; Spiegel & Foulk, 2006; Taras, 2005: Trost, 2007; Trost & van der Mars, 2010: USDHHS, 2008; USHR, 2008; Vail, 2006).

Engaging in physical activity:

- provides growth of new brain cells

- gives your brain a workout

- allows the body to improve general circulation

- increases blood flow to the brain

- increases the levels of norepinephrine and endorphins

- reduces stress

- improves mood

- provides a calming effect

- enhances synaptic activity in the brain or communication among brain cells

- leads to improved academic performance

- leads to increased attendance

- leads to decreases in health problems

- leads to less depression

- leads to engaging in fewer risky behaviors

Now, I am sure I missed a few, but you get the point, right? Ultimately, engaging in physical activity is very beneficial for your body, brain, and behavior. Who would *not* want to engage in physical activity, with all those benefits? Keep in mind (Beighle, Pangrazi, & Vincent, 2001), some children can test out as physically fit and not engage in any physical activity. However, chances are, if that person continues not to engage in physical activity over the years, their level of physical fitness will decrease. Unfortunately for children, especially those who lack physical activity in their daily lives, research shows (Schumacher & Queen, 2007) their role models do not engage in physical activity, making it hard for children to learn to be physically active.

Reports show (Pyle et al., 2006: Spiegel & Foulk, 2006; USDHHS, 1999) that approximately 50 percent of American youth aged twelve to twenty-one are inactive or lack regular physical activity. Typically, a life that continues to be inactive leads to a sedentary lifestyle. Unfortunately for many, a sedentary lifestyle has been a contributing factor to their death. Some may not engage in physical activity due to their environment. This may include a lack of parks or play areas nearby, safety issues, or the weather. However, numerous alternatives are available indoors or in safe environments. Alternative opportunities include hip-hop dance, yoga, high-intensity video gaming or small trampolines that can be used inside. Advocates of physical activity promote childhood as the key time to establish and begin to value the importance of regular physical activity (Cooper Institute, 2008; Prosser & Jiang, 2008; Vail, 2006).

Earlier I stated that the entire State of Texas began testing all students in grades three through twelve to determine how fit they were. How could this huge project, testing 2.6 million students, get started? In 2007 (TEA, 2008), an organization called Trust for America's Health published a report titled "Obesity Rates, % Children Age 10–17." At the time the report was published, the state with the highest number of obese children aged ten to seventeen was Mississippi, with 21.9 percent, or one out of five Mississippi students. In the report, Texas had the seventh-highest obesity rating in the United States among children aged ten to seventeen.

The state with the lowest percentage of obese children aged ten to seventeen was Oregon, the only state with a single-digit rating at 9.6 percent. Likewise, the top nine states had a rate of 20 percent or more, meaning one out of five children aged ten to seventeen in those states weigh in the obese range. As a result of this report, the State of Texas made physical fitness testing mandatory for all students in grades three through twelve, adding to the list of achievement testing areas in the state, to include reading, writing, mathematics, science, and social studies. The State of Texas decided to utilize the Fitnessgram to test the physical fitness of all those Texans. The following is part of the results from that study and a website is included in the notes section of this chapter where you can go to if your state is not listed or you want to know more.

Obesity Rates, % Children Age 10–17

Ranking	State	% of Children
1	Mississippi	21.9 (+/-3.5)
2	Georgia	21.3 (+/-5.1)
3	Kentucky	21.0 (+/-3.6)
4	Louisiana	20.7 (+/-4.0)
5	Illinois	20.7 (+/-3.7)

Source: Trust for America's Health, 2007

We have already discussed the results of the first year of Fitnessgram testing in Texas. In an effort to discuss data and research further, we are going to look at the second and third year of results now, which are showing some improvements. In addition, the number of students included in the research study is also growing. In the first year, there were 2,658,665 students tested; in the second year, there were 2,801,486 students tested, and in 2009–2010, there were 2,903,200 students tested. Still, all I have to say is, boys better get active! The complete three year results can be found in the appendices.

During the 2008–2009 school year, results were very similar (TEA, 2009). Once again, third graders tested out with the highest percentage of students in the HFZ. Again, third-grade girls tested out with the overall highest percentage of students in the HFZ. However, this year, the switch from girls testing with a higher percentage in the HFZ to boys occurred in tenth grade, as opposed to ninth grade. There were a few other points of interest I noticed, which included:

- Both years, third-grade girls had the overall highest percentage in the HFZ, with the first year tested being 33.25 percent and the second year increasing to 36.42 percent.

- Both years, twelfth graders, both girls and boys, had a single-digit HFZ percentage.

- Gains were seen at each grade level and for both girls and boys, with the exception of one year, eleventh-grade boys, who went from 12.24 percent the first year down to 12.16 percent the second year.

What does all this mean? If you have ten third graders, three, maybe four will probably test out as physically fit. In addition, for twelfth graders, maybe one of those ten students will test out as physically fit. However, before we leave this research study, I want to talk briefly about the third year of testing, which was during the 2009–2010 school year, when almost 3 million students were tested. Again, third-grade girls had the highest percentage testing in the HFZ; and again, the students testing in the lowest percentage were twelfth-grade girls. Also, again, both girls and boys in twelfth grade had a single-digit percentage of students in the HFZ. Yet, this time girls through tenth grade had a higher percentage testing in the HFZ. It just keeps getting higher and higher.

Physical fitness testing in Texas will continue and shows, *at each passing grade, the fitness levels decreased.* Percentages of students testing in the HFZ only started around 30 percent and went down every grade level, until the percentages were in the single-digit rates. National research (Pyle, 2006; Spiegel & Foulk, 2006; USDHHS, 1999) also follows this Texas research and shows as children get older, their level of physical activity goes down. In a press release (TEA, 2008, pg. 1), the founder of the Fitnessgram (the test utilized in Texas to test fitness levels of students) said, "We must immunize children against obesity while in elementary school, so that as they age, they are more likely to stay healthy and fit."

Are you beginning to understand how important being physically active is and why the fitness of students is being measured? From all this research, it appears we need to engage in physical activity on a regular basis. However, it does show now that students are being tested and working on increasing their physical fitness, positive changes are being made. I hope now that you know how important it is you too can make positive changes in your life. Let me tell you a story about Gina, who by age fourteen did not engage in much physical activity. I found the story of Gina as I was doing my own research (Puhl & Brownell, 2001), and this story really stuck out in my mind. I think it shows just how important physical activity really is. Gina was not very physically fit, and the results proved detrimental for her.

> TEXT BOX: But first ... how about a jumping jacks break. Do twenty jumping jacks, and get that blood flowing! Maybe even give your brain a workout!

Gina lived in South Dakota, was five feet four inches tall, and weighed 225 pounds. That means she had a BMI of roughly 38.4, placing her above the ninety-ninth percentile and in the obese weight-status category. Gina enjoyed writing poetry; she was an intelligent young girl and was even going to be skipping a grade in school. Unfortunately, Gina found herself in trouble. She had been caught stealing money from her parents and from lockers at school. Although she paid most of the money back, she was sent to a facility for petty theft. Gina said she stole the money to buy food.

Gina was admitted to a facility that treated low- to moderate-risk juvenile females for three to five months. Girls attending were to participate in a physical training component, which included a run between two to three miles. The facility realized the girls attending were not all physically fit; nor were students equally as physically fit as their peers attending the facility. According to the reports, it did not sound as if staff were very stringent or sticklers to any set rules on the two-to-three-mile, as staff at the facility allowed girls to fall out of the run or turn around prior to finishing the entire run, but staff encouraged all students to do their best. The goal was that by the end of the girls' time at the facility, they would be able to successfully complete the run. According to the operating memorandum of the facility, run by a former Marine, students were not to be pushed beyond normal training requirements.

One July morning, Gina began her run/walk. Upon Gina's enrollment into the facility, her physical fitness was such that she lacked the ability to complete even simple physical activities such as leg lifts, and her height and weight put her in the obese weight-status category. Early on, during the run/walk, Gina fell behind, and instructors attempted to encourage her in their own way. Ultimately, Gina collapsed; hitting the ground, and eventually an ambulance was called. Regrettably for Gina, it was all too late.

This does not mean all young, overweight teenagers (or people of any age) who engage in a two-to-three-mile run/walk will experience such tragic consequences. However, it does show the extreme consequences to a person who lacks physical activity and participates in physical activity at a high level. Mainly, I hope it affirms the importance of physical activity. In this section, we have talked about physical activity and about physical fitness, which tests a person's physical activity. We learned that a person who is not physically active could possibly test out as physically fit. We also learned that physical fitness typically decreases every year but we can stay active and *not* be a part of the statistics. We then learned about the many benefits gained by engaging in physical activity. We looked at a report on percentages of children aged ten to seventeen throughout the United States already considered obese. In addition, we looked at fitness rates of Texas students in grades three through twelve for the first three years, where students were mandated to complete fitness testing. Last, we learned just how serious the lack of physical activity can be in a person's life.

Now, we are going to look at the benefits that being physically fit provide you in school.

4.2 How Being Physically Fit Can Help You in School

Who would think being physically fit would really help you in school? There are many research studies regarding this very topic. Some of the information mentioned here may pertain more to being overweight or obese, which is what the lack of physical activity can eventually lead to (SSDHPER, 2005). In many cases, it is hard to differentiate if the problem is a lack of physical activity or if the students in a study are already overweight or obese, and as a result they are unable to participate in much physical activity, therefore causing them to lack physical fitness. Keep that in mind as you read.

Some researchers (CDE, 2002; Cooper Institute, 2008; Taras & Potts-Datema, 2005: Trost, 2007) Vail, 2006) feel the way to improve student achievement is by first considering how healthy the students are. When I first read that statement, I was amazed. As I continued my research, I realized just how true the statement was, and I am sure you will soon understand as well. In December 2002, the State of California announced the results of a study conducted throughout the state. The study (CDE, 2002) included physical-fitness testing using the Fitnessgram (as in Texas a few years later) and looked at comparisons between fitness scores and achievement in reading and math. The study included roughly 954,000 students in grades five, seven, and nine. Below are the four key findings resulting from this study:

- Higher achievement was associated with higher levels of fitness at each of the three grade levels measured.

- The relationship between academic achievement and fitness was greater in mathematics than in reading, particularly at higher fitness levels.

- Students who met minimum fitness levels in three or more physical fitness areas showed the greatest gains in academic achievement at all three grade levels.

- Females demonstrated higher achievement than males, particularly at higher fitness levels.

According to then-state superintendent Delaine Eastin (CDE, 2002, pg. 1), "This statewide study provides compelling evidence that the physical well-being of students has a direct impact on their ability to achieve academically." She went on to say the study provided them with the proof they had been searching for: "Students achieve best when they are physically fit."

A kinesiology professor at the University of Illinois conducted a study (Prosser & Jiang, 2008) and compared fitness scores to achievement in math and reading. The study included children ages eight, nine, and ten, as well as their BMI scores. The research findings revealed a strong relationship between math and aerobic fitness, meaning. students with higher BMIs had lower achievement scores, and students with higher aerobic fitness had higher math scores. So what is a relationship in a research study? A relationship (Creswell, 2008) is a way of measuring or describing variables. In this study, the variables were fitness scores and achievement. The researchers stated *healthier students are more ready to learn, and students with a higher BMI are not as fully prepared to learn.*

Now, let's talk about attention. We all know paying attention in class absolutely helps you in school. Scientists have noted that student attention is likely to be greater in active students as opposed to sedentary students (Vail, 2006). You may wonder about this, but if you go back and look at the long list of the benefits engaging in physical activity provides a person, it makes perfect sense that if your neurons are engaging, you are going to do better on a test than a peer with sedentary neurons. Additionally (Taras, 2005), if the blood flow to your brain is increased, you will probably learn better as well.

A group of scientists (Chomitz, Slining, McGowan, et al., 2009) who stated that student attention is likely to be greater in active students rather than sedentary students set out to gather data and determine if this was, in fact, true. Their study measured academic achievement in English and mathematics in fourth through eighth grade. Their sample, the group of students the scientists conducted their research on, included 3,990 students from a racially and economically diverse urban public school district in Massachusetts. The results found a significant relationship between a student's academic achievement and their physical fitness levels. There is that relationship in research again. It means the higher a student performed on the fitness test, the higher their odds of passing their achievement test.

Being physically active means *not* being sedentary, like a couch potato or a screen potato. A screen potato engages in a great deal of screen time—with things that have screens like a television, computer, video game, cell phone, or other electronic device that can make you sedentary. In recent years, there has been a steady increase in the hours spent watching television, the number of homes with multiple television sets, and even the numbers of cable subscribers and owners of VCRs, DVDs, and Blu-Rays. So, if there are more televisions and more cable and more ways to watch movies, then there are most likely more people engaging in sedentary activities, wouldn't you think? Additionally, while you are sitting or lying there engaged in screen time, you are being exposed to food advertising, increasing the urge to "munch." When you get the munchies, the desire for unhealthy junk food is more present than the desire for a nice salad, right? On the other hand, a healthy bowl of strawberries or carrots might satisfy your cravings. Keep in mind that engaging in screen time also takes you away from other things, like studying, or in many instances, sleeping. I bet at least once this week, you were texting when you were supposed to be studying, or playing on the computer or phone when you were supposed to be asleep.

One last research study I want to share with you, which also relays that the more fit you are, the better you perform academically, is my own research (Vaca Durr, 2010). I found it very interesting when I read statements saying the more fit a student is, the higher they will perform academically, so I set out to research this very statement. My research included fifth, eighth, and tenth graders in a Texas school district, a total of 1,545 students. I compared the fitness results from the Fitnessgram of the students with their test results on state achievement tests in math and science. In my research, I found that there was a correlation or a relationship between scoring higher on fitness testing and scoring higher on achievement in math and science. I also found in my research that younger students scored higher on fitness tests, and as students got older, few students tested in the HFZ. Now look at the following three charts as we talk about them:

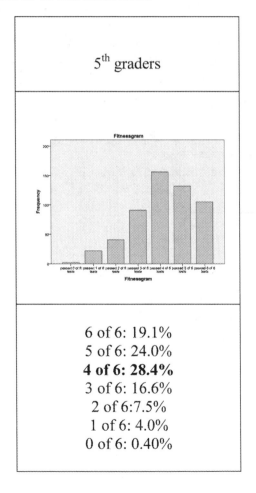

5th graders

6 of 6: 19.1%
5 of 6: 24.0%
4 of 6: 28.4%
3 of 6: 16.6%
2 of 6:7.5%
1 of 6: 4.0%
0 of 6: 0.40%

8th graders

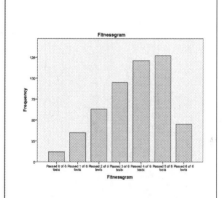

6 of 6: 9.0%
5 of 6: 25.5%
4 of 6: 24.3%
3 of 6: 19.1%
2 of 6: 12.7%
1 of 6: 7.0%
0 of 6: 2.4%

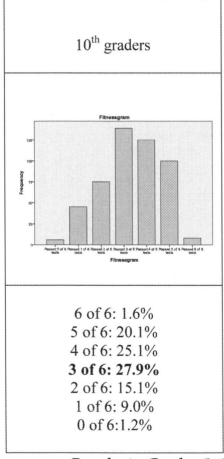

10th graders

6 of 6: 1.6%
5 of 6: 20.1%
4 of 6: 25.1%
3 of 6: 27.9%
2 of 6: 15.1%
1 of 6: 9.0%
0 of 6:1.2%

Fitnessgram Results in Grades 5, 8, & 10

The first column on all three bar graphs shows zero tests passed by students in that grade level. As you can see, the percentages of students at each grade level that passed zero parts of the Fitnessgram were very small. However, look how much bigger those percentages were in eighth (2.4 percent) and tenth grade (1.2 percent) compared to fifth grade (0.40 percent). Likewise, the last column on all three charts shows all six tests passed by students in that grade level, and again fifth grade has the largest column or percentage of students passing all six tests on the Fitnessgram, which was 19.1 percent. This means in fifth grade, about one out of five students passed all six tests, scoring in the Healthy Fitness Zone. By comparison, only 9.0 percent of eighth graders passed all six of the tests, and only 1.6 percent passed all six in tenth grade. I think this is a very large decrease. What do you think?

On the graph, there is one more interesting point worth noting, and I want to address this before we go on. When you look at the height of the columns, the columns appear to be tallest on the tenth-grade chart compared to the fifth-grade chart and even a little higher in eighth grade than the fifth-grade chart. Do not assume the numbers are higher in tenth grade, and even eighth grade, compared to fifth grade. The confusing part is answered on the left side of these charts, which is the frequency, going up and down. In fifth grade, the frequency goes up to 200, whereas in eighth and tenth grade, the frequency only goes up to 125. Therefore, the columns appear to be taller in tenth grade than they actually are.

Now, still talking about the bar graphs, look at the bottom row, where it states 0 of 6, 1 of 6, etc. That row shows percentages of students at each grade level who were able to master zero of the six tests given, one of the six tests given, all the way up to six of the six tests given. Then, in the box under the bar graph is another box with roughly the same information. By looking at the set of numbers in italics at each grade level, you will notice in fifth grade, the highest percentage of student scores on one test were four out of six tests at 28.4 percent. Then, in eighth grade, the highest percentage of student scores was five out of six tests at 25.5 percent and three out of six in tenth grade, with 27.9 percent. You can also look at and compare at each grade level how many students scored in the HFZ or mastered all six of the six tests, which goes from 19.1 percent in fifth grade to less than half that percentage in eighth grade, or 9.0 percent, and makes an even more dramatic decrease in tenth grade to 1.6 percent. I hope by presenting the information in more than one way, bar graph and written, the information was brought to life in a more helpful way so that you fully understand it.

We have just talked about how physical fitness affects you in school, and I hope the research and charts are making you think more about staying physically active and fit. We will talk more about this in chapter 5, where I will present a few more studies. Additionally, in this section, we talked about how being physically active benefits you. Now we are going to talk for a little while about those around you, like parents, family members, role models, culture, and friends affecting you. Again, remember I am not pointing the finger. We live in a culture that encourages eating more than enough and eating unhealthy foods. Keep in mind three goals of this book are to understand childhood obesity, to learn how *not* to become a statistic, and if you need to, to share the knowledge you gain from this book to help others learn the three goals as well.

4.3 How Do Those Around You Affect You?

This section is not about pointing the finger at others for causing childhood obesity. Rather, I want you to realize that others may not be doing you any favors, unintended or not. You need to realize that the actions of others could be negatively affecting you. Once you realize this, you are then able to say no or make a better choice for you. I always tell my children, "Their momma may say it is fine for them, *your Momma says no!*"

Did you ever hear about the lawsuit claiming McDonald's caused obesity? I will *not* tell you McDonald's causes obesity, and I hope you do not point the finger at them either. I will say that just like food from other restaurants, there are some foods on the menu that I will not eat or allow my kids to eat too often, but yes, I have eaten there before. McDonald's does not cause obesity; rather what *you* order, how often, and the amount *you* eat there could lead to your gaining a few pounds, just like food from other restaurants. It is up to *you,* not McDonald's; McDonald's will only serve what you order.

By saying that people around you may be affecting your weight, I am talking about parents, grandparents, relatives, and friends. Let's look at a few quick instances.

- You finish eating, feel full, and a family member next to you says, "I can't eat this all. Do you want the rest of mine?" You say no, but they beg you, and you eat it.

- You are told to finish your food but were given too much food to begin with.

- You do not have any fruits or vegetables during a meal, to snack on, or in a few days.

- You eat out, but your food is ordered for you, and you are not given options of healthier foods or healthier places to eat.

- Junk food is readily available and without restrictions (hard to say no).

These are just a few instances, and maybe you have encountered these in your life. Have you been in one of these situations before? I tell you about these so you can start to look for them, be aware of them, and have a plan and know how to handle them. Know that saying no (politely) is always a good option, as well as walking away or bringing your own bag of snacks. Maybe you can ask to take the extra food that you are unable to finish for lunch tomorrow or have it for dinner. In addition, ask your parents to buy fruits and vegetables when shopping for groceries and pack them as your snacks. Sometimes, if a parent is unaware you love kiwi or something you had at school, he or she does not know to buy it for the house. Moreover, they surely do not want to buy something and waste money because no one will eat it at home. Please learn to say "No thank you" when people offer you unhealthy foods, and start asking for healthier options. I know my Daddy always has bananas ready for my kids to eat when he knows they are coming.

In my research (AAAS, 2006), one other very interesting piece of information I discovered was how some cultures affect a person's weight, many times in a negative way. The most interesting articles regarding cultures and weight discussed how some cultures view a large family as an indication of wealth. By *large,* I am referring to the weight of the people in the family, not the number of people in the family. If the family members are large, it is proof that the head of the household is able to provide for the family. Reading this triggered commercials about starving children and how little they were, and it made some sense. Additionally, I recalled an episode of *The Biggest Loser,* when one of the contestants made a comment about his culture and weight. Think about the foods in different cultures and how too much of those foods (without a balance of healthy foods or physical activity) can lead a person to becoming overweight or obese. I know one of my favorite foods is enchiladas with rice and beans, and my Momma would make them every time I came home. If I came home too often, I would not fit into my clothes.

Before we leave this topic of how those around you affect you, I want to tell you a story about food, my Momma, and me. When I was in junior high and high school, I used to get sick a lot, and it actually took a few years before doctors realized I was not allergic to many foods, but rather I was very, very allergic to a ton of foods. It was not until I was in college that a doctor finally sent me to an allergist, after seeing many other specialists. I was actually going to the emergency room three to five times per month.

When I was younger, when I got up in the morning, my Momma made my breakfast, and I had some milk or juice. Unfortunately, we were unaware of the allergies at the time, and oftentimes I was actually allergic to the food and/or drink and would end up getting sick. My throwing up first thing in the morning always worried my Momma, and to this day I hate throwing up, but then who doesn't, right? There were many other symptoms besides having to get up from a huge table with tons of family to go throw up, such as pain in my chest that went down to my stomach, diarrhea, constipation, and nausea. After all this time, when we finally realized just how sick some foods made me, my Momma told me how bad she felt and how sorry she was. I had no idea what she was talking about, but she thought it was her fault I was getting sick, since she was the one who made my food. Although she was right, we were unaware of all the allergies, which were the real reason I was getting sick, but I was the one eating the food.

Nevertheless, it did trigger something in my mind as I began writing this section. During infancy and toddler years, our parents are directly responsible for the foods we eat: they buy the food, they prepare the food, and they give us the food. As we start getting a little older, they are still completely responsible for our meals, because they are the ones who buy the groceries. You probably have some say in what is purchased, because parents like to buy what kids like to eat and usually don't care to waste money on foods that will not be eaten. In my case, I was eating everything my Momma was making; we just did not realize *that* was the problem. As you get a little older, you need to know and learn about what you need to eat, what foods are healthy vs. unhealthy, and where you can go to get this type of information. Sometimes, the people who are responsible for our foods are not aware of the consequences of constantly eating unhealthy foods. Maybe they never learned about healthy versus unhealthy foods.

In this section, I hope you start to see that others may be negatively affecting your weight. This is a big step in learning to control your weight. In addition, by realizing that people around you or even your culture may cause weight gain, I hope you take measures to say no and make better, healthier options.

Chapter 4 Notes

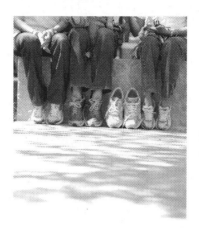

Source: jcannonphotography

DEFINITIONS

HEALTHY FITNESS ZONE (HFZ): A criterion-referenced standard, based on levels of fitness needed for good health, set specifically for boys and girls of various ages; not based on class averages or peer comparisons.

KINESIOLOGY: The study of the mechanics of body movements. What would a study of the mechanics of your body movement indicate?

ADDITIONAL INFORMATION

To find the entire report, Obesity Rates, % Children Aged 10–17, go to the following website:

http://healthyamericans.org/states/states.php?measure=overwieght&sort=data

TO DO

The following are role models I had growing up who participated in physical activity regularly:

- My Momma did aerobics at home with tapes and hand weights after we all went to school.

- My brothers were always very active in sports activities; my oldest brother was a physical training instructor for the Texas Game Warden Academy (talk about high-intensity aerobics).

- My sister married a man who trained/entered races (like marathons, half marathons, and 10k), which was an amazing moment for me as a child. Who knew people really did this stuff? Soon after, she started entering races, as did their children.

- My sister played volleyball and basketball in college.

List your personal role models who engage in regular physical activity. _____
_____
_____
_____
_____
_____

Who does the grocery shopping in your family? _____
_____
_____

Do you have any input in the groceries purchased? _____
_____
_____

If so, what do you add to the list? _____
_____
_____

Does your family have a weekly menu? _____
_____
_____

Do you think your family eats healthy meals? _____
_____
_____

Chapter 5: How All This Affects Me

If you are overweight or obese, you may or may not fully understand how this disease is affecting you. If you are not overweight or obese but have family or friends who are, again you may or may not understand the magnitude of this disease. Being overweight or obese affects a person in many ways, including many negative ways. Unfortunately, people often do not realize or think about the numerous negative effects. Even worse, some negative effects are unfathomable, and by this I mean most people will not believe an overweight or obese person has to put up with such negative behavior from others, including family members, classmates, educators, and sometimes even strangers. The effects of being overweight or obese are exactly why I am writing this book—so you, your family, or friends do not have to suffer the effects discussed in this chapter. Being overweight or obese can negatively affect a person:

- physically

- medically

- educationally

- socially/emotionally

Although we will discuss all four of these areas in some detail, many of them are intertwined; the results can negatively affect more than one area. In addition, keep in mind that being overweight or obese is not going to absolutely give you all these negative effects, and they will not negatively affect you immediately; it could be years before some occur, if ever. However, over time, these effects may occur, some quicker than others, some more than others, and some all at the same time. I am not saying the severity is all at a maximum level for every overweight or obese person, but slowly, these things may begin to occur. The first area we will discuss is physically, because just ten pounds overweight can start presenting problems.

5.1 How All This Affects *Me* ... Physically

The first area we will discuss is how childhood obesity or just being overweight affects a person physically. We will start by looking at what it means to be negatively affected physically because you are overweight or obese. For some people, this could mean getting sore from walking around too much, maybe even something as basic as walking from class to class. It can also include walking up and down stairs. Being negatively affected physically can also make a person tired faster and easier when engaging in physical activity, like walking to the next class. A person might be out of breath after engaging in physical activity, causing them to have to sit and rest awhile before they can finish their activity. Let's say you have the following morning schedule every day:

- walk to school—½ mile

- first-period math—on the second floor, back side of the school

- second-period computer—on the bottom floor on the other end of the school

- third-period PE—not too far past the computer class

- fourth-period science—back upstairs, across from the math class

- lunch—halfway back to the computer class

This may not look like a lot of walking, but say you only have five minutes between classes, and your locker is on the first floor, on the front side of the school. With a half-mile walk to school, and considering class locations, this could easily be a two-mile walk by lunchtime, with the large size of some schools. I used to work in a middle school and wore a pedometer. Most days, I walked four miles per day, sometimes even two miles before the first bell rang, and this was not even at a very large school.

Now, back to our school and schedule. If you throw in a fifty-minute PE class including suiting up, warming up exercises, about twenty minutes of a workout, a cool-down, and then getting cleaned up and dressed for class, this is a rough morning. What if, in class today, the PE teacher has you run two miles, or maybe play volleyball or run an obstacle course? You are going to be pretty tired by lunchtime, and if you are overweight or obese, chances are you will be worn out, possibly a little achy from PE class, out of breath, or late to your next class. In addition, the day still includes science, lunch, three more classes, and then a walk back home. As you can imagine, this student does not feel well, is very tired, and is losing interest in class. She nods off in science, as well as in the classes after lunch. Being overweight or obese is negatively affecting this student physically. The joints in her knees are hurting, maybe even her back; she lacks energy to get around, much less pay attention, and she is not happy throughout the rest of her schedule.

Affecting you physically includes causing you pain, discomfort, and aches that go with carrying around too much weight. Excess weight in children and teens is showing up as increases in bowed bones, altered gaits (the way a person walks or runs), as well as knee and hip pain. Now think of those infants we talked about earlier in chapter 1 who are not even walking yet but are already obese. Can you imagine how that extra weight is negatively affecting them as they *learn* to walk?

Years ago, I presented at a conference to parents regarding childhood obesity in a session titled *Are You Killing Your Kid?* I took a ten-pound block of fat with me, which I borrowed from the Extension Service. I asked any parents who had a child at least ten pounds overweight to strap the ten pounds on their back and walk the perimeter of the room, to experience what their children engage in on a regular basis. I had some parents almost fall over with the extra weight and many who were out of breath as they walked. One parent told me she did not realize how hard it was for her child to get around. I wanted parents to understand how hard it was for their kids.

In the next section, we will talk about how excess weight affects a person medically. This section will continue the discussion about physical effects.

5.2 How All This Affects *Me* ... Medically

Now we are going to talk about how being overweight or obese can affect a child or teen medically. Keep in mind, these effects are often shocking to people. They cannot believe these negative medical effects are caused by being overweight or obese. A major increase that has occurred due to being overweight or obese during childhood is in the number of children being diagnosed with type-II diabetes; a disease once seen only in adults (ADA, 2010). Today, type-II diabetes is affecting more and more young children. In addition, diabetes is the seventh-leading cause of death nationally (CDC, 2011), with death tolls even higher among some ethnic groups, including Hispanics and blacks. The sad part is that *type-II diabetes is a disease that is almost entirely preventable with a balanced diet and exercise.* It is not an easy disease to manage in adulthood, much less for a child to deal with.

Obese youth are also nine times more likely to have high blood pressure and are at increased risk of cardiovascular or heart disease, two more diseases typically not seen at young ages (AAAS, 2006). Another disease uncommon in children, sleep apnea, is occurring more frequent in obese children. One study (AAAS, 2006) indicated that 7 percent of obese children and 30 percent of very obese children suffer from sleep apnea, which occurs as a result of excess tissue in your neck, or muscle fat associated with obesity, causing your airways to collapse while sleeping. It could lead to heart failure or even death, which was the fate of a fourteen-year-old who weighed over three hundred pounds and died because of sleep apnea.

Research estimates that 50 percent of adolescent cases of gall bladder inflammation are related to obesity, as well as increased risks of polycystic ovary disease (AAAS, 2006). Increases are also occurring in children with asthma (Black, et al., 2012; CDC, 2011); by 2009, one in ten children had been diagnosed with asthma, with almost a 50 percent rise in black children being diagnosed. Overweight and obese children are also experiencing (CDC, 2011; Schwimmer, J.B., Burwinkle, T. M., & Varni, J. W., 2003; Taras & Potts-Datema, 2005) such medical problems as heart disease, arthritis, strokes, high cholesterol, nonalcoholic fatty liver disease, kidney failure, blindness, and neurological problems, not to mention increases in some cancers. Other medical problems include joint and circulatory problems, as well as pulmonary, gastrointestinal, and endocrine conditions—all diseases not typically seen in children at young ages or before graduating high school.

There are a few other medical effects, but we will discuss those in the social/emotional section. However, one more piece of research I came across often is very important, and I need to mention it before I leave this section regarding medical effects of being overweight or obese. Researchers point out that *once a person reaches adulthood and has already reached obesity, the probability is low that they will achieve an ideal body weight by engaging in voluntary weight loss.* That means most children or adolescents who reach adulthood, age eighteen, and already have a BMI in the obese range will find it more challenging to lose weight and decrease their BMI to a healthy weight, or for example, in an effort to reverse type-II diabetes. So, *increasing your physical activity and making healthier food choices is imperative for you and your friends or family members that are already overweight. Even if they are already in adulthood, you can help them!* But remember, it is up to *you!*

> TEXT BOX: Keep in mind, the research about being overweight by the time you reach adulthood does *not* mean there is no way you can get healthy again. Mainly, I write this to stress how important being

healthy is and to say it is much harder to *get healthy* than it is to *stay healthy!*

5.3 How All This Affects *Me* ... Educationally

The next section discusses how being overweight or obese can affect a child educationally, which many people do not think about. I will honestly say, even as an educator, I never thought about this. Remember the scenario we discussed at the beginning of this chapter and how being overweight or obese can affect a person physically. Do you remember all the walking the student had to do in school, just to get from class to class, not to mention the physical activity in PE class? Well, some of those negative effects are the start of negative educational effects as well.

I first realized that being overweight or obese could greatly affect a child's education negatively when I read an article regarding school days missed by overweight or obese students. The article stated (Schwimmer, J.B., Burwinkle, T. M., & Varni, J. W., 2003; Taras & Potts-Datema, 2005) that overweight or obese students miss, on average, four days of school per month. Again, being an educator, my mind started racing when I read this. It puzzled me more than anything. If school is in session only ten months per year, missing an average of four days of school per month equals forty days of school *per school year*. I don't know about all states or exact numbers of days that can be missed before a student will not be promoted. However, I do know the state I worked in only allowed ten days missed per year before a student would have to be retained (or make up those days). Therefore, this is very important and the start of eye-opening research for me. In addition, it means students will have to show up for Saturday school every weekend or be retained a few times. If a student can't show up on a regular school day, what are the chances they will show up on a Saturday?

Still remembering our student who was tired and out of breath by lunchtime, researchers (Vail, 2006) state that overweight or obese students have decreased energy to focus. In turn, this causes them difficulty with higher-level responses required for success in academics. I know when I am tired, I have a hard time focusing, especially in a class where the teacher is lecturing and has a very monotone voice, at which point you start dozing off.

Have you ever been around a person who suffers from sleep apnea? If you do not know what sleep apnea is, I have defined it in the notes section of this chapter, but real brief (AAAS, 2006), it is when airways collapse while sleeping. I have been in the middle of a very exciting and interesting conversation with a girlfriend who was diagnosed with sleep apnea. In no time, she was asleep! Another time, the worst part was, she was driving in the middle of downtown Houston traffic, and in a flash, she was nodding off, and I start freaking out. This is how serious sleep apnea is, and more children are suffering from the disease than ever before.

In class, what is that student who suffers from sleep apnea missing? They fall asleep in class and end up missing valuable lecture time, class discussion, and participation. You can imagine, if this happens on a regular basis throughout the day, this overweight or obese student is missing a great deal of class time in most classes. At this point, the student is physically in class, although he is experiencing the negative effects of being overweight or obese. Keep in mind, sleep apnea is uncommon in children; however, it is being diagnosed more frequently in obese children. Sleep apnea can also lead to death, in severe cases.

Research clearly documents that childhood obesity is leaving a negative mark on education. Being overweight or obese at such a young age can make a student lack concentration or focus during class (AAAS, 2006) because he is too tired from just getting from class to class. It may also leave an overweight or obese student with learning or memory problems as well. Additionally, many overweight students suffer from behavioral and social/emotional problems, which can also affect their grades in a negative manner. We will talk more about those issues in the next section.

You may wonder if there is any research supporting this theory. More and more researchers follow the concept that healthier students learn better. Fitnessgram creator Dr. Kenneth Cooper stated (Cooper Institute, 2008), "The more fit students are, the better they will do in school, while students that are overweight lag behind at each grade level." Departments of Education in California and Texas began testing the physical fitness of their students and comparing physical fitness to academic achievement. Results in both states indicate that in fact healthier students *do* perform better academically.

At this point, you may be thinking about an overweight friend you have who makes straight A's. I know a few people in school as well that were overweight but still very smart. Keep in mind there are those very smart students who are not physically fit and are not physically active. The research states overall, a fitter student will learn better. Remember we talked about the Texas fitness testing results, which included all students in grades three through twelve and began during the 2007–2008 school year? We also discussed other research that stated as people get older, their level of physical activity decreases, which is why staying physically active now is so important. We want to be smart enough for college when we get there too.! Next, we are going to talk about how being overweight or obese affects a person socially and emotionally.

5.4 How All This Affects *Me* … Socially/ Emotionally

This section addresses the negative ways childhood obesity affects a person socially and emotionally. I must warn readers that this section was very painful to write. As I was doing my research, I was flabbergasted by the stories I read. Before we get into some of the stories, as always, we will first talk about the research and then discuss the research and the stories included.

Researchers write that children suffering from childhood obesity suffer a great deal of emotional pain, have a decreased self-esteem, and suffer a high risk of depression and eating disorders (Schwimmer, J.B., Burwinkle, T. M., & Varni, J. W., 2003; Taras & Potts-Datema, 2005). Obese children also experience increased psychiatric disorders such as anxiety, stress, loneliness, and depression; are more likely to be victims of bullying, experience increased behavior problems, and are more vulnerable to alcohol and drug abuse. In addition, research indicates they experience emotional pain, are perceived as less desirable by peers, have a distorted body image, and are excluded in many social situations.

I remember when I was in second grade, at age seven, at Tyler Elementary—a few years before iPods and iPhones—an over-aged, obese boy named Manuel sat in front of me in this grumpy old teacher's class. I know for sure Manuel was very overweight and may have been in the obese weight-status category. I am not sure, as I was just seven years old. I also think he was older than I was, but I am not sure how much older. I do know that Manuel was so big, he did not fit in a regular second-grade desk, so he sat at a round table with a chair.

As I remember, for some reason, the teacher made me his personal assistant. I had to sit at that big table with him and help him read and do class work. I was so little at Manuel's bigger table, my feet did not reach the floor. At recess, nobody picked Manuel to be on their team for Red Rover because he refused to run and really could not run too fast; when he did, classmates would make fun of him. Sometimes Manuel would even fall when he tried to run or his pants would start falling down. In addition, no one would pick me, because I was too small and short to reach the line, much less break through the line. So here we were, Mutt and Jeff, teased and excluded. I remember when we were made to run, Manuel was always very tired when we got to class, and unfortunately, that grumpy teacher would pop his hand with a ruler when he fell asleep. Thinking back, it's no wonder Manuel missed so many days of school. As his personal assistant, I always felt bad for him.

Self-esteem is largely developed during childhood, as a result of experiences encountered. A healthy or positive self-esteem, for example, comes from experiences such as being praised; being allowed to talk and actually being listened to; being spoken to respectfully by family and others; getting attention and affection; and experiencing success, such as in school or extracurricular activities. As you can imagine, a low or negative self-esteem develops as a result of opposite experiences, including being harshly criticized, ignored, ridiculed, teased, yelled at regularly, and even beaten. In addition, self-esteem can be damaged by expecting to be "perfect" all the time or to do the right thing and from experiencing repeated failures, such as in school or extracurricular activities. As you can imagine, it is hard to keep your head up when all these negative experiences are going on around you, especially when the experiences are occurring at home *and* at school.

What do you think are the consequences of low self-esteem? The consequences include anxiety, stress, loneliness, and negative self-image, increased likelihood of suffering from depression or experiencing problems with both friendships and relationships. Research also shows (Strauss, R. S., 2000; Taras & Potts-Datema, 2005) consequences of low self-esteem can lead to low academic achievement and an increased chance or participating in risky behaviors, such as alcohol and smoking. Now let's think about Manuel for a minute. If he never had any successful experiences on the playground, fell asleep in class often, and was publicly punished in class, and was already overage and behind in school, how low do you imagine his self-esteem was? I just cannot imagine.

Think about this as I retell other stories I found in my research. Often, people experiencing poor self-esteem rely on current feelings—how they are feeling *right this minute*. If situations are going positively, their self-esteem could be rising; if situations are more negative, their self-esteem could continue to fall. However, if they already feel bad on the inside, how can the outside be good (outside meaning happy, smiling, cheerful, fast-paced, etc.)?

You may wonder if overweight and obese children really do have low self-esteem and how researchers were able to determine this. Research shows (Puhl & Brownell, 2001; Schwimmer, J.B., Burwinkle, T. M., & Varni, J. W., 2003; Teachman & Brownell, 2001) children themselves, some as young as nine years old, report their self-esteem is low. They believe the reason they are teased, do not have as many friends as peers, or are not picked for teams and sports is because of their weight. *In America, research states* (Renck Jalongo, 1999) *the number one reason for peer rejection is being overweight.* Junior high (or middle school), and high school, as well as just being a teenager is hard enough on any child to begin with, but then adding low self-esteem and peer rejection is way too much for any child, youth, or even adult to handle. Unfortunately, the fact is, this does not start in later years; studies show these behaviors begin at very early ages.

One study (Puhl & Brownell, 2001) conducted in 1961 and replicated for roughly twenty years and in different cultures showed that even children as young as four years old rejected obese peers. Further research indicated that obese children were, and continue to be, negatively stereotyped by healthy-weight children. It also stated, "Obese persons are the last acceptable targets of discrimination." For the overweight and obese student, it is hard to believe they would even show up to school knowing their day will be full of pain and suffering, just trying to get around. Not to mention the suffering they also have to deal with, as well as ongoing prejudice, unnoticed discrimination, and a great deal of constant harassment and rejection throughout the day on a daily basis.

Some people even publicly ridicule overweight and obese children and youth in restaurants and stores for their food choices. Recently, I experienced a similar type of ridicule for food choices I was giving my two sons. My daughter and her Daddy went out on a very special military event for Princesses and their Hero's, their military Daddy! I decided Momma and the boys (ages four and two) would go out for a fun night. Our plans immediately took a detour, due to horrible weather. After an hour of messed-up plans, our only option for any fun was that I had rented a great movie at the library that the boys watched in the truck, while eating a bag or carrots and cucumbers. The only dinner option was to go back to the base restaurant near the house. When I informed the boys of the altered plans, they immediately stated they wanted a grilled cheese and some applesauce. At this point, they did not know I was going to surprise them with something special, especially since the night was proving to be not so special.

Now, so you don't have to assume anything, like the woman who came to our table and made a negative comment, let me say that my boys had already eaten three fruits that day (two for breakfast and one for lunch) and four vegetables (two for lunch and two in their snack bag in the truck). This was a very typical day of fruits and vegetables for them. In addition, at the time, the boys weighed thirty-three and thirty-seven pounds and had a BMI of fifteen to sixteen, which is a healthy number. The final surprise was a cup (measured, one full cup, not more, not less) of ice cream! I believe it was the first time in his life my two-year-old had ice cream (unless my parents or sisters had given him some and I was unaware). The boys were in heaven when the waitress brought the surprise, and I could tell by looking just how much they enjoyed it!

Then a woman came to our table and asked if she could get some napkins from the dispenser on our table, because her table didn't have any (although there were empty tables closer that did have a napkin dispenser that she could have just taken). I said "sure," and the boys, still enjoying their ice cream, asked her name. She never gave her name, but said, "Don't you think you boys need to be eating your vegetables?" I almost choked on the sip I had just taken, got up out of my chair, and said, "Excuse me?" She looked at me and said, "Shouldn't they be eating their vegetables?" At that moment, there were so many things running through my head, and I could not help but think *who does she think she is?* When I continued to stare at her without speaking or sitting down, she finally just walked away. Keep in mind, this woman was *not* at a healthy weight by any means. At best, she was in the obese range (past overweight). At the time, my boys were in a healthy range, and I was probably still a little overweight. There were so many things I wanted to say, but my parents always told me not to act like a fool, and I usually try to abide (most of the time).

As we walked out, the woman tried to continue a conversation with me, but I remember my little niece, when she was about to get in trouble, saying, "Walk away, walk away!" and that really helped! I tell you this story to show how pretentious and intrusive people can be and for no good reason! They assume something and then take action on their assumptions, making a fool out of themselves by opening their mouth.

Research shows overweight and obese children suffer exactly this type of discrimination on a regular basis. They are often considered (Puhl & Brownell, 2001; Teachman & Brownell, 2001) lazy, lacking willpower, sloppy, unattractive, and less successful. The reality is, they are often completely opposite of these descriptions. Before we leave the topic of how being overweight or obese can negatively affect a child or youth's self-esteem, let me tell you another story. I found this story with the National Education Association (NEA, 1994), and will say I was crying by the time I finished reading it. The girl experienced outrageous behavior throughout her childhood and adolescent years. It was stated that she never had any friends and was ridiculed and bullied every single day. You may think the worst part of her day was when she walked down the halls and boys flattened themselves against lockers while hollering "wide load." In fact, this was not the worst part of her day.

She felt the worst part of her day was at lunchtime and the apparent production it provided her peers, as she was eating her lunch. The girl did everything to avoid the cafeteria: hide in bathrooms, behind gyms, and throughout the school, inside and out. Hers is a brutal story that no child or person of any age should ever have to live through. One day, schoolmates started throwing food at her while she was seated at a table. She says *plates* of spaghetti splashed onto her face, and long, greasy strands dripped onto her clothes. She goes on to say everyone was laughing, pointing, and making pig noises. All she could do was sit there. The story does not say if she was overweight or obese, merely that she was not at a healthy weight. I cannot imagine experiencing such outrageous behavior and then realizing this was a daily experience she had to endure.

I do not know any more about this girl—her weight, if she had any medical issues, or her demographic data, like age, grade level, etc. However, I can almost promise she was experiencing three if not all four (physical, medical, educational, social/emotional) of the negative effects associated with being overweight or obese. Unfortunately, she experienced these negative effects throughout childhood and adolescence.

Have you ever been around when peers were teasing or bullying an overweight or obese student who walked by? What did you do to help? Did you help the overweight or obese student? Or did you participate in the ridicule? The girl in the story said she never had any friends. Can you imagine going through childhood and adolescence all alone, with no friends? Maybe you can try to be a friend or at least stop the outrageous behavior.

Research shows the reason most people act like such fools is that they fear they could one day become overweight or obese, (Puhl & Brownell, 2001) just like the person they are ridiculing. If you are overweight or obese, I am very sorry if you have ever had to experience such outrageous behavior. I pray you can go on to the next chapter and get the tools you need to make positive, lifelong changes. A very good friend of mine had a daughter in seventh grade, and one summer she vowed she was tired of being overweight and was going to lose those unwanted pounds. She was very determined, and in three months over the summer, she was at a healthy weight. Therefore, I do know it can be done (or at least significant changes can be made), and I am rooting for you! In addition, we will talk about what you can do in the next chapter.

Chapter 5 Notes

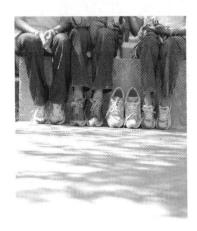

Source: jcannonphotography

DEFINITIONS

TYPE-II DIABETES: A form of diabetes that usually occurs in people over forty years of age but may develop in younger people, especially in minorities. Most people who develop type-II diabetes are insulin-resistant. However, some simply cannot produce enough insulin to meet their bodies' needs and others have a combination of these problems. Many people with type-II diabetes control the disease through diet and exercise, but some must also take oral medications or insulin. (*http://www.americandiabetes.com/ resources/diabetes-glossary#t*)

SLEEP APNEA: A common disorder in which you have one or more pauses or shallow breaths while sleeping, lasting from a few seconds to minutes, often occurring thirty times or more an hour. Typically, normal breathing resumes, sometimes with a loud snort or choking sound. Sleep apnea usually is an ongoing (chronic) condition that disrupts sleep. When breathing pauses or becomes shallow, a person will often move out of deep sleep and into light sleep, making the quality of sleep poor, making one tired during the day. Sleep apnea is a leading cause of excessive daytime sleepiness. The most common type of sleep apnea is obstructive sleep apnea, meaning the airway has collapsed or is blocked during sleep, causing shallow breathing or breathing pauses. Obstructive sleep apnea is more common in overweight people but can affect anyone, for example, small children with enlarged tonsil tissues in their throats. For more information go to: *http://www.nhlbi.nih.gov/health/health-topics/ topics/sleepapnea/.*

SELF-ESTEEM: Self-esteem is the belief that you are important or valuable. It is not that you think you are perfect and better than everyone else. It is more like thinking you are worthy of being loved and accepted. If you want to read more, go to: http:// kidshealth.org/kid/feeling/emotion/self_esteem. html. Examples of experiences that provide high self-esteem include: being praised; being treated with caring and warmth; experiencing success;

and parents spending time with their children. Examples of experiences that provide low-self esteem include: being called names; being treated harshly; never experiencing success; or parents speaking in hateful or ugly terms.

ADDITIONAL INFORMATION

As I wrote about schools and all the walking, I got a little curious and wanted to know a little more, so I called a good friend of mine named Ward Hughling, who is a coordinator for construction services. That means he works with the builders that build new schools for a school district. I asked him two questions, and his answers were very interesting, at least when you think about physical activity. My questions were, "What is the average size of middle schools and high schools in the district?" and "Considering the average size, if you walked the entire school, inside (first and second floors), how many miles would it be?" He quickly answered (which surprised me) with the following average square feet and termed my second question as "walking the corridors":

Average size of middle schools: 117,500 square feet or 1.25 miles if you walk the corridors.

Average size of high school: 314,000 square feet or 2.50–2.76 miles if you walk the corridors.

Now, I realize not all schools are this big. Remember that middle school I mentioned working at? It is actually approximately thirty thousand square feet smaller than the average size mentioned above. However, I still walked many miles each day. I hope this does help paint a picture.

If a student cannot make it to school on a daily basis, how can we expect they will be able to make it to Saturday school every Saturday? However, if they miss an average of four days per month, they would need to be there *every* Saturday.

KEY POINT

Keep in mind, just because you may be an overweight teen, that does *not* mean you have to stay this way; nor does it mean you will automatically become an overweight adult and you cannot get healthy again. You *can be at a healthy weight again!*

Chapter 6: What Can I Do?

We have shown that *childhood obesity results from an imbalance in physical activity and caloric intake.* Therefore, it is reasonable to think that *the key to weight loss is the opposite—increase physical activity and decrease caloric intake.* However, the right balance of healthy foods, or caloric intake, is also extremely important.

The Key to Healthy Weight

**Increase
physical activity**   **Decrease
caloric intake**

If you look around, you will soon notice that there are hundreds of diets on the market, but we are not going to get into any specific diets. However, I will share a secret to weight loss that I have found many people, including me, simply *disregard.* The secret to shedding those unwanted pounds is *honesty,* being completely honest with the most important person in your life; not the doctor, not your parents, not your friends … being completely honest to *yourself!* You have to be honest about everything that goes into your mouth and every bit of physical activity you engage in. You have to be honest about the keys to being healthy for life. After all, if you say you ate an apple for breakfast and only took a bite and then dumped it for a bag of chips, are you really being honest? In addition, the worst part is you are only lying to yourself! If you cannot be truthful to yourself, whom can you be truthful to? For this reason, I say *honesty* is a necessity for weight loss and therefore the secret to a healthier weight.

In this chapter, we will talk about adding physical activity to your daily schedule and caloric intake. Then we will talk about a plan to help get us on track and shedding those unwanted pounds and becoming healthy for life. Basically, we will be talking about the key to healthy weight or how to balance our scale.

The Secret to Weight Loss ...

Being completely honest with yourself about everything regarding your caloric intake and your physical activity!

Honesty!

6.1 Adding Physical Activity to Your Daily Schedule

First, let's make sure that we fully understand the title of this section. Yes, the title does say *Daily Schedule,* not "once in a while schedule," not "once a week schedule," but every single day. Now that we understand what *daily* means, research shows

(AAAS, 2006) that long, long ago, people used up much more energy on a daily basis than is typically consumed today.

Have you ever heard your grandparents say they walked five miles or more to school, one way, uphill, in the snow, barefoot … and the story just goes on and on regarding their hardships in getting to school each day? The story may have some truth to it and unquestionably, many embellishments. Nevertheless, the story does make an excellent point regarding physical activity in the lives of our ancestors. Have you ever seen the old television show *Little House on the Prairie* (my favorite childhood show) or maybe *The Walton's* and noticed how much physical activity the characters engage in on a daily basis? You can still catch re-runs of both shows. The characters walked to the store, to school, to church, to play, to the barn; basically, they walked almost everywhere they went. On rare occasions, they rode on a horse and buggy, but typically not on a regular basis, and usually only when they had goods to haul.

The point is that the characters engaged in a great deal of physical activity. Think how much you would walk on a weekly basis if you had to walk to and from school every day and to the store every time you needed something; to practice, to the game, and to church. In addition, if you ever went shopping or to a friend's house to hang out or out to eat, that would just add more miles. Actually, why don't we just calculate how many miles you would walk in a week if you were to walk everywhere you went?

I am going to list a few places you may go on a weekly basis. On the space next to it, write down the roundtrip mileage; then add all the miles for your weekly grand total. I also left a few extra spaces for other places you may go during the week. I left room on the left for you to write how many times you go. Then on the right, write the weekly grand total.

For example, if it is a two-mile round-trip walk to school and you go five days a week, you will write 2 (in the blank on the left) to school; x 5 = 10 (on the blank on the right).

- _____ to school; _____
- _____ to the store; _____
- _____ to church; _____
- _____ to practice; _____
- _____ to visit grandparents; _____
- _____ out to eat; _____
- _____ to hang out with a friend; _____
- _____ to a game; _____
- _____ to the library; _____
- _____
  _____

- _____
  _____

- _____
  _____

So what is your weekly GRAND TOTAL _____?

When I completed my chart, I came up with 64 miles of physical activity in one week and that did not include any workouts, runs, or going to visit any family or friends. These 64 miles merely included taking my kids to school and practice, going to the grocery store and running errands, and taking my kids to games, the library, and movies. Now do you understand how people in the days of *Little House on the Prairie* examples were more active? I don't know about you, but I am sure I would have to sleep more compared to what I do now, leave earlier in the morning than I do now, and I might not be too interested in playing ball or going out to eat, especially if it was too far. I sure would not want to visit many family or friends too often, if it was very far.

People during these times used up a great deal of energy in their daily lives. They also did not participate in a great deal of sedentary activities, because—well, actually—most sedentary activities that we know today had not been invented. On *Little House on the Prairie,* they did not have television, Xbox, Wii, cell phones, computers, Blu-rays, or "i"-anything. Therefore, they could not sit and be "couch potatoes." Even in later years, past *Little House on the Prairie* days, when there was television, there was not an overabundance of channels available, nor did channels go twenty-four hours per day. In addition, fast food was not readily available (depending on how many years we want to go back). In some cases, people had to hunt for food in the wild, the stream, a field, the henhouse, a slaughterhouse, or any number of places. As you can imagine, there was a great deal of physical activity included in people's lives "back in the day."

With developments in transportation, fast food, and technology, we have become a much more sedentary culture, resulting in a decrease to our amount of daily physical activity. A large majority of children and youth today do not walk or ride their bike to school, they are driven; additionally, they are driven to and from extracurricular events, church, the store, shopping, and to a friend's house. When they forget until ten minutes prior to bedtime that they need a poster board for class tomorrow, they are driven to the store to pick it up; they do not walk. Now please don't think I'm being judgmental; I often drive to the store that is a quarter mile away from my house if I have too many items to purchase or the items I am purchasing are too heavy. It is a lot easier to walk to get bread, cheese slices, some Band-Aids, and a roll of paper towels than it is to walk to get a gallon of milk and a honey-baked ham.

The point in all this is that the changes that have occurred over time are exactly why physical activity has been taken out of our daily schedule. Adding physical activity to our daily schedule is extremely important if we (yes, me too) are going to decrease our current weight to a more healthy weight and live healthy for life. In addition, if you are reading this book to help a friend, family member, or even yourself, the way to start is to get up and get moving, either on your own or with the friend or family member you are trying to help. One important note to make before we get started on increasing physical activity: if you, your friend, or family member is very obese and does not participate in any physical activity at this time, they might need to be checked out by a doctor first. *Initially, we need to make sure you (or whomever) are healthy enough to participate in physical activity.* However, do not allow this to become an excuse for not starting to engage in physical activity; get that appointment made immediately.

Now that we have talked about a few changes that have evolved in recent years, we are going to talk about how to get started getting physically active. Do you remember when you were in elementary school and your teacher had you keep a reading log every day? In it, you wrote down how many minutes you read each day, and your parents signed off, ensuring you did in fact read those minutes? Each week, you had a goal of about twenty minutes per day, and if you had an awesome teacher like Mrs. Chris Curtis and Mrs. Beverly Hansen, you received a prize at the end of the week for reaching your reading goal. The reason your teacher had you read is because research shows daily reading improves your reading ability.

So, what is a physical activity log? Basically, a physical activity log is much like a reading log that includes all of the physical activity you participate in for a set period of time. It includes a specific time period, a place to write how much physical activity you participated in on each day, and includes notes—for example, how you felt after an activity or how much fun you had. It also includes goals and indicates if they were achieved. When I finally realized I needed to get healthy for life, I came up with the idea and used it for myself. As a former teacher who gave out those reading logs, I thought this would be a great way to see a few things regarding how I was doing. The physical activity log told me:

- How I am doing each day, week, month;

- How I am progressing. For example, it may have taken eighteen minutes to walk a mile when I first started, and in a month, I was down to fifteen and a half minutes;

- Specific goals, for example, at first I was just trying to walk two miles four times a week, but as time went on, I was able to add miles and days, and if they were mastered; and

- The log helped kept me focused and motivated to continue.

The following is my initial physical activity log:

Physical Activity Log for (week): _____

Sun.	Mon.	Tues.	Wed.	Thurs.	Fri.	Sat.

NOTES: _____

_____

GOALS	ACHIEVED
1) Work out 4 days per week	
2) Work out at least 20 minutes each time	
3) Try 30 minutes at least once	

Source: Vaca Durr, 2012

As you get more and more physically active, your goals will change, ultimately achieving sixty minutes per day, seven days a week. The point is to keep up with all your physical activity. As you write in your log, be sure to make any notes on how you felt, especially if the activity you engaged in hurt or made you feel sick. Of course, if you are not physically active, when you start, your body will get sore, but *it should go away in a few days … keep on!* Remember how we talked about the secret to shedding those pounds and how we need to be completely honest. Please make sure when you write in your physical activity log, you are completely *honest.* For example, if it was a quarter mile, do not write a mile or even a half-mile. You are only being dishonest with yourself. Over time, you will be able to see improvement, I hope. In addition, by keeping notes, you will know how you felt at times, if you got hurt, and when it was very hot outside. In addition, your goals will change with time; *keep challenging yourself.*

Research provides us with the following number of minutes needed daily to start burning stored fat, to stay at a current weight, and to lose weight. The chart is listed below; however, I do not want you to think that you need to go from being inactive to the maximum number of minutes in a week. Rather, you need to build up to the appropriate time gradually.

- 20 minutes: Your body will use up active calories, not the stored-up calories where the fat is stored.

- 30 minutes: At a moderate intensity, your body will stay at current weight.

- 60 minutes: At a moderate to vigorous intensity, your body will lose weight.

Keep in mind, if you, your friend, or family member has completed a physical activity log baseline (that first week worth of physical activity data when you start) and is only able to complete ten minutes, four days a week without a problem, then we will not start out with seventy-five minutes of physical activity per day. If you are at ten minutes, four days per week, maybe your goal should be ten minutes, seven days per week. Once you are able to do that without problems, increase your time to twelve minutes, and then bump it up to fifteen minutes one of those days. However, if you are already at twenty minutes per day, seven days per week with no problems, try thirty minutes, two days per week and twenty the remaining five days. Small increments will make it easier on your body but still help you get to where you want to be!

Also, *do not start making excuses!* If it is raining or snowing outside, do not start the excuse game, saying, "Oh, the weather is too bad to work out!" *Do not allow weather, or forces outside your control, to become your excuse not to work out, ever!* Bad weather just means you need to be creative and find alternative places to work out or alternative workouts. Go to the mall (but stay focused on walking, *not* shopping), march in place in your bedroom (or anywhere) the entire time (it will be like walking on a treadmill … you are walking but not getting anywhere, just burning calories), or walk inside your school or church before you come home. Be sure when someone asks what you are doing, you stress that you are getting healthy for life or doing your daily exercise. *You never know when you might motivate someone else to join you.* They could be using the same excuse you considered using and could benefit in joining you or benefit from your motivation and willpower not to allow any excuses to stop you from participating in physical activity.

As you begin to add physical activity to your daily schedule, be on the lookout for ways you can add activity that is even more physically challenging into your already busy schedule. Let's face it: sometimes just finding the time to exercise can be a chore in and of itself. If your parents drive you to school, ask them to drop you off half a mile from the school or even a mile away. As you are able to do the walk easier, have them drop you off farther and farther from the school. Just make sure you get to school.

Other ways to include physical activity into your daily schedule could be to take the dog for a walk (or if you don't have one, take the neighbor's dog); walk to the store when your mom needs some whole-wheat bread; play hide-and-seek with your little cousin; or even dance (not slow dancing). You could also play soccer or baseball with your little brother, push your cousin on a tricycle, rake the fall leaves, or shovel the winter snow, no not with a snow blower. You could also mow your grandma's yard (front and back) and help her pull the weeds, go swimming, or push the cart when your parents go to the wholesale food store and buy a ton of healthy foods. I know from experience, pushing that cart with two children in it gets heavy!

When you have completed your activity, make sure you add it to your physical activity log, along with the number of minutes spent. You may think gardening does not include physical activity. It might surprise you. On our last move, I had a big, weed-filled yard. One day I spent pulling weeds, bending over, sitting here, and moving there for three hours. The next day, I was very sore, and I am typically rather active; I am just not weed-pulling active, apparently. Even working out on a regular basis, you use different muscles for different types of physical activity, like pulling weeds, which can make even an active person sore in different spots.

This brings me to another topic we need to talk about: types of physical activity your workouts should include (AAAS, 2006). These three areas are similar to those listed in chapter 4, which included aerobic, muscle-strengthening, and bone-strengthening, and offers some suggestions you may enjoy. Again, if you are not currently physically active, *DO NOT* start all of this in week one. Gradually work up to becoming physically active, and know that your workouts should eventually start including the following three categories:

1. Cardiovascular conditioning: this improves your heart health and burns the most calories. This category includes physical activity such as running, biking, and swimming.

2. Stretching: this improves your flexibility. This category includes activities such as stretching,

yoga, or tai chi. You could also add pulling weeds, which includes a lot of stretching.

3. Resistance training: this improves muscle strength and endurance. This category includes activities like weight training.

Now, let's talk about this first before you go out and buy some weights. When we talk about weight training, the weights do not have to be actual weightlifting weights, especially if you have never lifted weights in your life. Actually, if you (your family members or your friends that you are helping) are just getting started, *do not go out and buy any weights yet.* First, go to the pantry or the cupboard, where the canned food is stored. Do you see any eight-ounce cans, such as tomato sauce? Grab one of those in your hand and drop your hand to your side. Hold on tight to the can; it will hurt your toe if you drop it (ask me how I know). With the can in your hand, lift it straight out horizontally. Do that twenty times with each hand, with the can in your hand. This can be your introduction to weight training.

Then do some curls with the can. For curls, your arm is in front of you and curl your arm up (toward your head) and back out to a level position. Do that twenty times with each hand, with the can in your hand as you do them. How did that feel? I know, you felt silly in the kitchen lifting tomato sauce, seems like a strange place for a workout, but this is a perfect place to get started. If you have never lifted weights, you sure do not want to go straight into the gym and try a bar with twenty pounds on each end. Your arms may be sore tomorrow, yes, from the eight-ounce can.

Nevertheless, you will get used to it, and before long, you will be promoted from an eight-ounce-can lifter to a fifteen-ounce-can lifter, or from a tomato sauce to ravioli, and eventually to a twenty-two-ounce-can of beans! Be careful to hold on tight to the can, so you don't drop it or throw it while you are lifting. And don't go too fast; that also increases the chances of dropping or throwing the can across the room. (Unfortunately, I know this by experience.)

We have discussed how changes have caused a decrease in daily physical activity in today's age and how much physical activity you would get if you had to walk everywhere you went. Then we talked about physical activity logs, what is included in a weekly log, and how the log can help monitor progress as your physical activity increases. A physical activity log can also help us show progress as we increase our daily physical activity and meet our weekly goals. Then we talked about the three areas of physical activity you need to include in your routines, including cardiovascular conditioning, stretching, and resistance training. I hope you give a great deal of thought to starting with that eight-ounce can of tomato sauce and work your way up to big cans of beans before you go out and buy weights or a gym membership. Now we are going to talk about the other part of balancing our scale, the caloric intake.

6.2 Our Caloric Intake

In this section, we will talk about our caloric intake, including foods and drinks that need to be included in our daily menu. We will also include those it would be beneficial to *decrease* from our daily menu. We will also talk about benefits of different-colored foods, you know like red foods, green foods, etc., as well as reading labels and portion sizes. We will learn the differences between portion sizes and serving sizes and will end this section by talking about a weekly caloric intake log.

I hope you have heard we should all *eat five to seven fruits and vegetables per day.* Unbelievably, some people do not eat *any* fruits or veggies any day. That is a way to keep from losing weight and even get clogged up, preventing healthy bowel movements. Many years ago, I spoke at a conference and said, "You should eat a rainbow every day," meaning you should eat something that represents each color of the rainbow every day. A first grader at the conference with his mother heard me make this statement and took it to heart. He made sure he held himself and his mother accountable to this statement. Together they tried to include a rainbow in their diet every day.

This is a great way to get started balancing your scale, by making sure you eat fruits and vegetables every day and trying to include all the colors in the rainbow in the colors of your fruits and vegetables. What might a rainbow in your diet include, or what would it look like? Let's look at a rainbow, the colors that are included, and list a few fruits and vegetables for each color:

- **Purple:** grapes, plums, blackberries, raisins, eggplant, purple cabbage, onions, passion fruit, mint flowers, mulberries, lavender

- **Blue:** blueberries, juniper berries, blue grapes, blue potatoes, cauliflower

- **Green:** spinach, kiwi, broccoli, cucumbers, celery, bell peppers, grapes, zucchini, avocado, apples, asparagus, brussels sprouts, cactus, chives, collard greens, fennel, green beans, olives, honeydew, kale, lettuce, limes, mint, okra, swiss chard, tarragon, tomatillo

- **White** (I know, white is not a color of the rainbow, but some people say you need white foods ... so pretend you see white in the rainbow): onions, bananas, cauliflower, mushrooms, coconut, jicama, shallots, turnips, garlic, horseradish, buckwheat, tofu

- **Yellow:** corn, squash, pineapple, nectarines, apples, anise seed, bamboo shoots, lemons, parsnips, pears, saffron, yellow tomatoes, summer squash, star fruit

- **Orange:** carrots, peaches, oranges, cantaloupe, butternut squash, mangos, orange peppers, papayas, winter squash, tangerines, sweet potatoes, persimmons, pumpkin, apricots

- **Red:** watermelon, raspberries, cherries, radishes, tomatoes, apples, strawberries, cranberries, grapefruit, guava, red cabbage, red peppers, tomatoes, rhubarb,

You may be wondering why a rainbow needs to be presented on your plate daily and what, if any, nutritional values these different-color foods may have. Different-color foods do have different nutritional values. Here is a graphic regarding the nutritional values of various fruits and vegetables, based on color (which includes white, which is why I added it to our previous list):

- Purple foods: promote microcirculation

- Green foods: rejuvenate musculature and bone

- White foods: enhance immune system, lymph system, and cellular recovery

- Yellow foods: optimize brain functions

- Orange foods: support skin and mucosal tissues

- Red foods: support heart and circulatory

After looking at all the great benefits various colors of fruits and vegetables provide you, who would not want to eat a rainbow each day? Hold on, I think I need a yellow food break! How about you join me?

A great source to help you get on the right track to eating healthy for life is *www.mypyramid.gov*. When you go to the website, you enter your age, gender, and your current amount of physical activity. After entering all the information, you will be supplied a food pyramid specifically for you that states the amounts and types of foods you should be eating daily. The categories include:

- grains

- vegetables

- fruits

- oils

- dairy products

- low-fat meats and beans

Each category is represented by a color, and you will notice each color is a different width, depending on how much of that category you need daily. The great thing about the website is it is specialized to you and it is free!

A successful meal plan combines eating fewer calories and eating balanced meals. When counting calories or how much from each category you consume daily, also keep in mind how much you drink. You just might be surprised how many calories, how much fat, sugar, etc. are included in some drinks. It might be even more surprising how just taking sodas out of your daily diet will improve your health and possibly drastically decrease your caloric intake. Also, be sure to drink the appropriate number of ounces of water per day, *each day!* I know, drinking too much water makes you have to go to the bathroom a lot. I thought that too when I first started drinking sixty-four ounces of water per day. It gets better the longer you do it; at least it did for me.

Water is good for you; it helps hydrate you, removes waste, and protects your vital organs. You should drink forty-eight to sixty-four ounces of water each day (AAAS, 2006). When I started drinking all my water daily, I was *running* for the bathroom, what felt like every fifteen to twenty minutes. At first, it was like a chore, one of those dreaded chores you hate doing. At the time, I was working in an extremely fast-paced environment, and running to the bathroom every fifteen or twenty minutes was *not* always an option. I was an assistant principal at a middle school and had what felt like a revolving door of referrals. When I broke up my water, it made it easier for me to handle. By putting it in measurable containers and spacing them out throughout the day, I was able to get all my water in daily and not have to worry too much about running to the bathroom at the most inappropriate time. I broke my sixty-four ounces up as follows:

- 12 ounces on the drive to school

- 24 ounces throughout the school day

- 12 ounces on the drive home

- 16 ounces when I got home

Figure out what works for you and your schedule, and don't forget to measure it out so you know it is sixty-four ounces! And a word to the wise: scope out all the bathrooms before you get started; it just might come in handy! Make sure other liquids, such as juice or sodas are *not* added as water; they are *not water* and do not count.

On the other hand, and not to be a party pooper, carbonated drinks are really not so good for you. You knew that already, right? Research shows (Malik, Schulze, & Hu, 2006) the odds of becoming obese increase with each can of sugar-sweetened beverage consumed. Carbonated drinks are high in sugar, and many are high in caffeine. They have practically no nutritional value, and many contain inappropriate additives and are not considered part of a healthy diet. In addition, many drinks provide up to three servings in one container, meaning they are so big, one could actually make up three drinks.

This leads to two other topics we need to talk about in this section: learning to read labels and portion sizes. Eating is like adding fuel to a vehicle. Food allows your body to run, just as gas allows your vehicle to run. What happens when you put regular gasoline into a vehicle that requires diesel fuel? If you put a few ounces in a tank, you will be fine, but if you *fill that tank* with diesel, or the wrong fuel, then your vehicle just will not run. *Eating unhealthy foods in small amounts and not on a regular basis is also fine, but when you fill your tank with the wrong foods, your body will eventually just not run right.*

Now we are going to talk about reading labels, those that appear on the backs of food products, specifically written "Nutrition Facts" on the label. You might even learn why junk food is called junk food, but I am not going to talk too much about that, because I have a feeling you know about junk food.

What do those labels on the back of food products say? Let's look at a label or Nutrition Fact and find out. If you have never looked at one, it will be a great learning experience for you. The bullets on the right or outside of the box in our example tell you what you need to check for when looking at the nutrition facts of foods and drinks. The first two lines give you the serving size and the number of servings in this one box or bag. This is important, because there are probably times when you eat a whole bag and are not even aware that the bag was two or more servings. Make sure you pay attention to this section!

The next section is very important, as it gives you the number of calories per serving. It also tells the amount of fat, saturated fat, cholesterol, sodium, total carbohydrates, and protein. This section is great for helping you keep track of how many calories or other nutrients you are getting from a specific food. The remaining parts of the Nutrition Facts state the percentage of daily value in the food and are also very helpful. Please make sure to read all this information in the box below and use it as a tool in planning your meals or what you choose to eat and eliminate. For more information, you can go to *http://teamnutrition.usda.gov/Resources/read_it.pdf.*

Product:

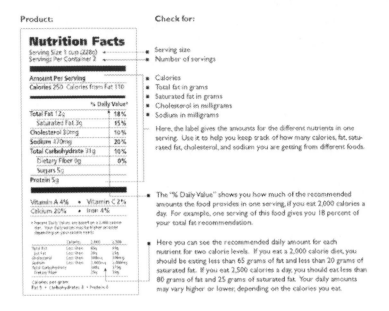

Check for:

- Serving size
- Number of servings

- Calories
- Total fat in grams
- Saturated fat in grams
- Cholesterol in milligrams
- Sodium in milligrams

Here, the label gives the amounts for the different nutrients in one serving. Use it to help you keep track of how many calories, fat, saturated fat, cholesterol, and sodium you are getting from different foods.

The "% Daily Value" shows you how much of the recommended amounts the food provides in one serving, if you eat 2,000 calories a day. For example, one serving of this food gives you 18 percent of your total fat recommendation.

Here you can see the recommended daily amount for each nutrient for two calorie levels. If you eat a 2,000 calorie diet, you should be eating less than 65 grams of fat and less than 20 grams of saturated fat. If you eat 2,500 calories a day, you should eat less than 80 grams of fat and 25 grams of saturated fat. Your daily amounts may vary higher or lower, depending on the calories you eat.

Source: CDC

By knowing how to read the nutrition facts or the label on foods, you can see where to make changes and cuts, and which foods to run from. Also, be on the lookout for healthier options for foods like salad dressing, hamburgers, or your favorite foods. Look at foods like carrots, pickles, or plums, all great snacks usually with few calories.

Do you remember in the first section of this chapter when we talked about the number of minutes of physical activity needed daily to start burning stored fat (twenty minutes), stay at a current weight (thirty minutes), or lose weight (sixty minutes)? One pound of fat equals 3,500 calories.

I went to *www.choosemyplate.gov*, and after inputting a little bit of information, I had a Daily Food Plan developed for my great niece, my kids call her "Iguana!" but her name is really Gwynneth. A copy of the plan is below, and I thought it would help us in this next section.

My Daily Food Plan

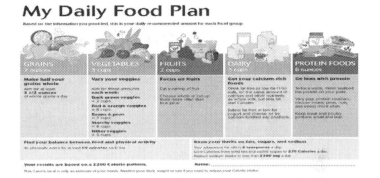

Source: CDC

The information I had to enter included height, weight, age, sex, and level of daily physical activity. The chart gives the exact amount of grains, vegetables, fruits, dairy, and protein needed daily, stating results are based on a 2,200-calorie diet. Now that we know Gwynneth requires 2,200 calories per day, in order for her to lose weight, she could either increase her physical activity or decrease her caloric intake. Say she wants to lose one pound per week; she could either burn 3,500 calories per week by working out or cut 3,500 calories per week from her diet, or a combination of the two.

But first, we have to know how many calories per week she is eating. Much like the physical activity log, she needs to determine how many calories she is consuming before she can look at the above guidelines and lose a pound per week. However, determining your daily caloric intake is a starting point, and then you can go from there, because you will have your baseline data, similar to increasing your daily physical activity.

If you discover you eat much more than 2,200 calories per day, then the first goal will be decreasing your caloric intake to a healthy level, *although not by making a huge change overnight.* For me, when I realized my physical activity and caloric intake scale were totally out of whack, I started reading labels and keeping track of everything. I realized it was harder to decrease my caloric intake than to add physical activity, and before long, I was looking for ways to make healthier choices. This is when I discovered light ranch dressing and turkey burgers, and then realized how much I already loved mustard and pickles to begin with!

Writing this information down—physical activity and caloric intake—is a great way to keep you accountable for it all and to keep you honest to yourself! Below is a chart I use. We can call it a caloric-intake chart; I call it a weekly calorie chart. The notes section of the chart is used to write down foods you eat often, along with the serving size and their calories. When you write the information down, you will see where all the calories are coming from, and you may want to tweak your daily diet or even make some huge changes in some areas. I know one thing I realized is that if I am going to have a snack at night, I need to either plan for it beforehand or I need to change my nightly snack (yes, to pickles). In time, you will be able to make some positive changes toward being healthy for life.

Caloric Intake Log			
Sun.	**Mon.**	**Tues.**	**Wed.**
B-fast: _____ ___	B-fast: _____ ___	B-fast: _____ ___	B-fast: _____ ___
Snack: _____ ___	Snack: _____ ___	Snack: _____ ___	Snack: _____ ___
Lunch: _____ ___	Lunch: _____ ___	Lunch: _____ ___	Lunch: _____ ___
Snack: _____ ___	Snack: _____ ___	Snack: _____ ___	Snack: _____ ___
Dinner: _____ ___	Dinner: _____ ___	Dinner: _____ ___	Dinner: _____ ___
Snack: _____ ___	Snack: _____ ___	Snack: _____ ___	Snack: _____ ___
TOTAL: _____	TOTAL: _____	TOTAL: _____	TOTAL: _____
Thurs.	**Fri.**	**Sat.**	**Notes:**
B-fast: _____ ___	B-fast: _____ ___	B-fast: _____ ___	B-fast: _____ ___
Snack: _____ ___	Snack: _____ ___	Snack: _____ ___	Snack: _____ ___
Lunch: _____ ___	Lunch: _____ ___	Lunch: _____ ___	Lunch: _____ ___
Snack: _____ ___	Snack: _____ ___	Snack: _____ ___	Snack: _____ ___
Dinner: _____ ___	Dinner: _____ ___	Dinner: _____ ___	Dinner: _____ ___
Snack: _____ ___	Snack: _____ ___	Snack: _____ ___	Snack: _____ ___
TOTAL: _____	TOTAL: _____	TOTAL: _____	TOTAL: _____

Source: Vaca Durr, 2012

Portion sizes is another topic we need to talk about before we start developing our plan toward being healthy for life. You need to be aware of it as you try to decrease your caloric intake. Do you remember the website we talked about with the specialized daily plan just for you (*www.mypyramid.gov*)? The specialized plan also lists the amounts of food from each category that should be consumed daily. The example for my niece Gwynn stated that daily she needs to consume:

- seven ounces of grains,

- three cups of vegetables,

- two cups of fruits, three cups of dairy, and

- six ounces of protein

The plan even states she should aim for six teaspoons of oils daily, half of her grains should be whole grains, and it breaks down her vegetables, stating that over the course of a week, she should try to get the following:

- 2 cups of dark green vegetables;

- 6 cups of orange vegetables;

- 2 cups of dry beans and peas;

- 6 cups of starchy vegetables; and

- 5 cups of other vegetables

The website even has a site where you can track both your caloric intake and daily physical activity, so it might be worth walking to the library to check out. It gives out cool reports, tracks everything for you, and does most of the work.

What exactly are portion sizes and serving sizes? I went to the United States Department of Agriculture (USDA) website (*http://www.cnpp.usda.gov/Publications/NutritionInsights/insight11.pdf*), where I found a definition. According to the USDA, *a serving size is a unit of measure used to describe the amount of food recommended for each food group.* For example, the previous chart shows a serving size equal to one cup. To find the recommended amount of food, look on the Nutrition Facts or label. A *portion size,* on the other hand, *is the amount of food eaten and can be as big as you choose* (which is where you need portion control). Therefore, it is very important that you understand the difference between serving size and portion size and document it correctly.

If you go to a buffet and write down that you ate chicken, corn on the cob, broccoli, and an apple, to determine how many calories you consumed, you need to know how much of each item you ate. To determine how much you ate or how many servings you ate in your portion size, you need to get into the habit of weighing and measuring your foods; otherwise, how will you know if you ate a cup of broccoli or if you ate six ounces of meat? Do not get confused between serving size and portion size.

Before we leave this topic of portion sizes, I want to mention that portion sizes appear to have grown a great deal over the last twenty years, no pun intended. A cheeseburger at a fast-food joint twenty years ago was roughly 330 calories; today it is almost 600! An order of spaghetti and meatballs included a cup of spaghetti, about three meatballs, and came to about 500 calories, whereas today an order of spaghetti and meatballs is over 1,000 calories.

Being from Texas, I have seen Texas-size orders and boy, those calories are high. (I think there are even calories just smelling some of the food!) The important thing here is not only keeping track of the portion size but also keeping *control* of those portion sizes. Often one of the best things to do is order a to-go box when you order your meal; that way, at least you can spread your calories over two meals. Again, being aware of this will help you on your journey to being healthy for life. In our next section, we will be putting all of this together and developing a plan so you, your family member, your friend, or whomever can be healthy for life.

6.3 A Plan to Help Get Us on Track ... Just for You!

Now that we know what causes childhood obesity, the key to weight loss, how much physical activity we need daily, foods we should consume, the amount of water we need to drink daily, and reading labels, serving sizes, and portion sizes, it is time to put all this knowledge together and put it into action. We need to develop a *doable* plan just for you—or whomever you might be trying to help. What is a doable plan, and how is it different from just a plan? I want a plan that will work for you, a plan that will help you (or your friend or family member) go from where you are today to a successful healthy-for-life lifestyle, making it doable and therefore assist you in your journey toward becoming healthy for life.

To get started, I am going to make a list of four things for you to consider before we start developing your plan. Each point will include a question you need to ask yourself and some you may need help with. I added a bit of information after each question for you to think about. I will try to give you some resources along the way, so you aren't wondering where to go for help. The following are the four questions and the bit of information you need to think about before you get started (with room for any notes):

1. *Are you healthy enough to get started, or do you need to be checked out by a doctor first?*

     THINK ABOUT: If you have any medical problems or are very overweight, a doctor should check you out first. If you do not know if you need to be seen by a doctor before starting your road to healthy for life, go ask your school nurse. If you do need to go to the doctor first, tell the doctor what your plan is, and see if he or she has any suggestions, restrictions, or advice to offer.

_____

_____

_____

_____

_____

_____

2. *How much physical activity do you currently participate in on a daily basis?*
   THINK ABOUT: Remember the physical activity log we talked about? If you do not know how much physical activity you participate in, start that log today for a week. If you cannot remember everything you did today, that is fine; just write what you are sure you did. In a week, you will have your baseline and can go from there. Keep up with it daily.

_____

_____

_____

_____

_____

_____

3. *What is your daily caloric intake?* That includes everything that goes in your mouth. Be honest!
   THINK ABOUT: Tomorrow morning, start your caloric-intake log, including *everything* that goes into your mouth. When you are finished, you will see which areas need work and which areas you are doing well. Start

measuring your foods. You might be amazed what an appropriate serving size is and looks like up close and personal.

_____

_____

_____

_____

_____

_____

4. *How are you coming along with the daily H_2O?*
   Or are you just getting used to the information?
   THINK ABOUT: Start keeping track of your daily water intake. Also, look for the best times to drink your water. During or before you start a meal is always a good time.

_____

_____

_____

_____

_____

_____

It should take about a week, maybe ten days for you to gather all your baseline data and other information to answer the four questions above. I promise, the planning will pay off in the end and help you increase your success. The more you know about this new, healthy-for-life lifestyle, the higher the chances you will be successful. It is kind of like taking a test: the more you listen in class and the more you practice, the higher the chances you will make a good grade. In case you are wondering what else you could be doing in those seven to ten days while you are gathering your information and baseline data to help increase your success, I have a list of things you can be thinking about or doing. I know, you're so happy, right? Can you tell I like lists? Here is the list of the things you can be thinking about or doing in the next seven to ten days while you gather the information from the last list. I have also broken the list down into sections, to help you understand each section in more detail.

1. Think about ways to add physical activity into your life.

2. Go on a grocery store field trip.

3. In your schedule, where can you find time to add activities involving your new lifestyle?

4. What about breakfast?

5. What about your shoes?

6. Junk food and sodas (and other items you can cut from you caloric intake)?

6.3.1 Ways to Add Physical Activity

Think about ways you (or your friend or family member) can add physical activity into your life. I know I gave you some ideas, but I want you to think of some doable ones just for you and write them down. There may be a rock-climbing wall down the street from your house, a swimming pool, or a skating park—all ways you can add physical activity into your life. You may enjoy dancing or Zumba, so add that! Just make sure you aren't slow dancing but rather working up a good sweat. Now write about six options for you. Make sure they are physical activities that you enjoy.

List Six Physical Activities You Enjoy

1._____

_____

_____

2._____

_____

_____

3._____

_____

_____

4._____

_____

_____

5._____

_____

_____

6._____

_____

_____

6.3.2 Grocery Store Field Trip

Go on a field trip. Yes, a field trip, to the grocery store or a farmer's market. Walk through the produce section, where all the fresh fruits and vegetables are located. On your field trip, you are going to make a few lists. In addition, as you look around, see if the grocery store has placed recipe cards or nutritional value information near some of the produce. Take the cards and read them. It will add to your knowledge, as you begin your journey to your new healthy-for-life lifestyle. You could also take a friend or parent to enjoy the experience with you. They may learn something too, and you both might have a positive experience that will help you be successful in your new lifestyle. If you go with the right attitude, an attitude of interest while gathering knowledge, it should be fun. Here are the three lists you are going to gather on your field trip:

1. Fill in your rainbow—list a few fruits and vegetables for each color that you like (and therefore plan to eat).

2. List three to five new fruits you are going to try—write down three to five fruits you have never eaten before but you are going to try on your new journey.

3. List three to five new vegetables you are going to try—write down three to five vegetables you have never eaten before but you are going to try on your new journey.

I added an example to give you a visual (keep in mind, my choices are limited due to allergies):

Green

> Fruits I LIKE: grapes, apples, kiwi, limes
>
> Veggies I LIKE: spinach, zucchini, bell peppers, avocados, broccoli, chives
>
> Fruits I will TRY: sweetsop (also called sugar apples)
>
> Veggies I will TRY: okra, brussels sprouts, cactus,

- Purple

  o Fruits I LIKE: _____
    _____

  o Veggies I LIKE: _____
    _____

  o Fruits I will TRY:_____
    _____

  o Veggies I will TRY: _____
    _____

- Blue

  o Fruits I LIKE: _____
    _____

  o Veggies I LIKE: _____
    _____

  o Fruits I will TRY: _____
    _____

  o Veggies I will TRY: _____
    _____

- Green
  - Fruits I LIKE: _____
  _____

  - Veggies I LIKE: _____
  _____

  - Fruits I will TRY: _____
  _____

  - Veggies I will TRY: _____
  _____

- White
  - Fruits I LIKE: _____
  _____

  - Veggies I LIKE: _____
  _____

  - Fruits I will TRY: _____
  _____

  - Veggies I will TRY: _____
  _____

- Yellow

  - Fruits I LIKE: _____
    _____

  - Veggies I LIKE: _____
    _____

  - Fruits I will TRY:_____
    _____

  - Veggies I will TRY: _____
    _____

- Orange

  - Fruits I LIKE: _____
    _____

  - Veggies I LIKE: _____
    _____

  - Fruits I will TRY: _____
    _____

  - Veggies I will TRY: _____
    _____

- Red

  o Fruits I LIKE: _____

  _____

  o Veggies I LIKE: _____

  _____

  o Fruits I will TRY: _____

  _____

  o Veggies I will TRY: _____

  _____

6.3.3 Finding the Time

One big problem you may encounter with your new healthy-for-life lifestyle is finding the time for various activities you will be adding to your new lifestyle! Instead of time becoming an obstacle for you—and ultimately an excuse—let's talk about what I mean when I say, "finding the time." At first, you may think this new lifestyle is a bit time-consuming, which is why I am pointing this out to you at the beginning of your journey. Always remember, first of all, this is a new lifestyle, and it will include some changes. Once you are used to those changes, it will become much easier, and you will find ways to cut that time whenever possible. At first, it will require some time on your part. Here are a few things that will take some time out of your normal schedule but will still be worth the new lifestyle:

- Participating in daily physical activity

- Weighing and measuring your foods

- Cooking healthy foods (as opposed to eating fast food)

- Recording your data

- Extra visits to the bathroom

When will be the best times for all these activities? The best way to find time to add these activities is by first seeing if there are any activities during your day that you can eliminate or spend less time on, so you can add one or more of your new lifestyle activities. Sorry, but this doesn't include schoolwork or homework! Have you considered eliminating some screen time or doing your new lifestyle activities during commercials? Next is a chart for you to complete listing when you will do the following activities, along with some suggestions on where you may find time that might be beneficial to you as you get started:

New Activity: Participating in daily physical activity

> My Suggestions: Whenever it is best for you; maybe as soon as you wake up or right when you get out of school.

Your Plan: _____
_____
_____
_____
_____
_____
_____
_____

New Activity: Weighing and measuring your foods

> My Suggestions: It is easier to wash/chop/bag a cup of fruits or vegetables when they come home from the grocery store. Then, in the morning just grab and go.

Your Plan: _____

_____

_____

_____

_____

_____

New Activity: Cooking healthy foods

> My Suggestions: You may not be the family cook, but helping is a great way to learn how to help make healthier food. Remember, this is a new "forever" lifestyle, so you will be using these talents forever!

Your Plan: _____

_____

_____

_____

_____

_____

_____

_____

New Activity: Recording your data

> My Suggestions: Immediately after you do it, that way you do not forget, and the data is more accurate.

Your Plan: _____
_____
_____
_____
_____
_____
_____
_____

New Activity: Extra visits to the bathroom

My Suggestions: Quickly! Waiting too long may be bad for you.

Your Plan: _____
_____
_____
_____
_____
_____
_____
_____

I have never been a morning person, so working out first thing in the morning has always been worse than sitting through a boring class with a monotone teacher. I usually work out right after work or school, although now it is more when it fits in my children's schedule. Before participating in your physical activity, keep in mind how far you will walk or run or whatever you do and how long it will take so you can better plan.

Regarding time, another area you may need to find time for is packing your lunch. You should pack lunch either first thing in the morning or at night, right before you go to bed. Another block of time you might want to look at is sedentary time—when you are sitting and watching TV, surfing the Internet, or off in la la land oblivious to things going on around you. Sitting in class is *not* sedentary time. While you are watching TV, maybe you could add some stretching or get those tomato sauce cans out and start your "can lifting" routine. I sometimes watch the news while I walk on the treadmill. Think about it: if you are going to just sit there and watch TV for an hour, it is the perfect time to add some physical activity, don't you think?

Be on the lookout for ways of adding what you need to your schedule. Never give the excuse, "I don't have time," when you have been sitting there watching TV or surfing the Net. One other point I want to stress before I leave this topic is regarding preparing food. It used to take a long time for me to cut up all my vegetables for a salad or cut up my apple during the day. I started cutting up the vegetables when I came home from the grocery store with them. Then I would store them in containers or bags of one serving size. The night before, I would grab a container of veggies, a container of fruits, or I would put a salad together, put everything in my lunchbox, and it was ready for the morning. The next morning when I woke up—especially if I woke up late or spent too much time looking for something to wear—it was easy to just grab my already-packed lunch when I rushed out the door.

I would also pack my water, so it would be cold and ready. I would then figure out what I was going to have for breakfast and get it ready too. When I ran out the door, I would have my lunchbox, water containers, some coffee, and my breakfast. Yes, I ate my breakfast in the truck on the way to work, but I had a forty-minute drive. Find what is best for you.

Look at the following schedule. Take into consideration your homework, the time, and your schedule. You have roughly two hours to get about an hour's worth of homework completed and your daily physical activity marked off your to-do list. Here is a sample schedule and list of activities:

> **4:00**—You get home from school, have a snack, and have the following homework: about thirty minutes worth of math, an essay to type, and a science project to start on.

> **6:00**—Dinner.

> **6:45**—Leave for practice.

> **7:00–9:00**—Choir practice.

> **9:15**—Return home; shower; finish homework; pack lunch for tomorrow.

> **10:00**—Get ready for bed.

If this were my schedule, I would do the math homework first, and immediately after I was done, I would change clothes or put my walking shoes on. (It would be about 4:35 or 4:40 when I was finished with all this.) Then I would quickly type up a rough draft of my essay and save it to come back to later; it would be about 5:00. Since I am already ready for practice, I would go straight to the park, walk for thirty-five minutes, and then walk home. It takes five minutes to get there, plus thirty-five minutes of walking, and five minutes home, so it should be about 5:45. I have fifteen minutes to either shower or review my essay before printing; if I'm quick, I could do both and be ready for dinner at 6:00. When dinner is over, you have time to help clear the table and get your stuff out to start on your project for a little while when you get home. Alternatively, you could pack your lunch. The more organized you are with your schedule, the easier it will be to get everything done. I usually try to schedule my workouts, and I often have to tweak that schedule, but when I at least have an idea of when I'm going to work out, it is easier to include in my schedule.

6.3.4 What about Breakfast?

Breakfast is very important because it offers nutrition for your brain. It is also a perfect time to add some fruit or vegetables to your diet. Grab an apple, cut it in quarters, and eat it on the way to school. If you'd prefer, even a handful of cherry tomatoes will be good. If you grab both the apple and cherry tomatoes, you could be one fruit and one vegetable for the day down and only three to five left. Grab a bagel and an apple or some yogurt; grab some grapes or a cucumber or strawberries, some oatmeal or even a breakfast bar (make sure it really is healthy). You could also grab two slices of bread, put some peanut butter on one, jelly on the other, and then cut up a banana and put it on one side and have a nice PBJ with bananas sandwich, as my son says, "That is YUM E for my tummy!" Be creative; just make sure you have breakfast.

You may be one of those people who does not like breakfast, although it is fuel for the brain, and you do want that brain fueled up! Breakfast does not have to be eaten immediately after you wake up, nor does it have to be an elaborate meal. On your road to a new and healthy-for-life lifestyle, start trying to make it a daily part of your day to have breakfast, even if it is at 9:00. Before you know it, you may just love it. In addition, it may give you the extra push you need to get to your goal weight, and that can't be a bad thing. I know I enjoy oatmeal and a piece of fruit most mornings, because oatmeal is good for my cholesterol and I have inherited bad cholesterol. So there can be more benefits to eating breakfast than just fueling your brain, which is a really big one to begin with.

6.3.5 What about Your Shoes?

The next thing I want you to think about is what shoes you are going to be wearing while you participate in physical activity. While this doesn't mean you should go tell your parents you need a new pair of shoes, you *do* need to walk in a good pair of athletic shoes. A good pair of walking shoes needs the following:

- a low, stable heel

- a flexible toe

Eventually, as you increase the amount of walking or physical activity, you will need to invest in a pair of shoes that provides a little more support, is better on your feet, and used solely for workout purposes.

One thing to keep in mind is that your feet get bigger while you are working out. I went to a running store, so they could fit me for a pair of walking/running shoes, about a year after I had gotten into exercising on a daily basis. My feet, normally size five, expand two sizes while I walk or run, and I ended up leaving the store with a size seven shoe, which shocked me! I cannot do anything else with those shoes but work out in them, otherwise I look like a clown. If you know of a running store near you, take a field trip there and check it out. While you are there, you can also look at prices and start saving. If you are not serious about this new healthy-forever lifestyle, maybe you do not need to invest in an expensive pair of shoes; but if you are serious, a good pair of shoes will help you immensely. However, in the meantime, a good pair of insoles will go a long way too.

The employees at most running stores are often avid runners who have a wealth of helpful knowledge regarding running, starting a running program, and running events like 5Ks, half-marathons, and marathons. I'm not saying you should try to run a marathon (and NO, I have never run a marathon), but I am saying a 5K would be a great goal to add to your list. At some point after you feel you are ready, try one out. There may even be some walking or running events held at your school. Be on the lookout for these, and if they scare you now, just put them on the back burner. You can also volunteer at a large running event such as a half-marathon or marathon, just for the experience. By being a volunteer, it will help you know what you are getting into before you decide it is something you want to do.

6.3.6 Junk Food and Sodas

We all know chips, sodas, pies, cakes, donuts—all that stuff that really makes you go mmm-mmm—really is not good for you. I will merely ask you to read the labels on those things and tell me if there is anything healthy about them. I know you are not going to avoid them for the rest of your life, and I admit I have not either. A healthy-for-life lifestyle does *not* mean I will never buy and consume junk food again. I do not, however, have them readily available in my house so I can use them as an excuse when I get hungry or when I get upset, stressed, or overwhelmed. Instead, I buy them when I know we have a special day or event, and they will be eaten quickly after they are purchased. Sometimes I use them as my reward for meeting my weekly physical activity goal, but I *do* add them to my caloric intake.

Look at junk food and sodas as a way of celebrating your achievements as you begin your journey to a healthy-for-life lifestyle. I predict that eventually, on your own, you will start having healthier foods for your celebrations, with more thought going into the celebratory foods. And don't think it was fast-food restaurants that made America fat, as we said before; it was Americans that chose to order the food that made them fat. Don't go blaming someone else, and don't let anyone else blame a restaurant or food; we all make the choices of what goes in our mouths. Now it's time to make a list. In this section, I want you to fill in the following information:

Go look in the pantry or cupboard (where all the dried foods are stored). What junk foods are there? _____
_____
_____
_____

Which *one* is your favorite? _____
_____
_____
_____

How many calories and carbohydrates does it have? _____
_____
_____
_____

What is the serving size? _____
_____
_____
_____

How long could you go without having it? Could you go a day? Two days? How about until you reach your first goal? How about having it once a month?_____
_____
_____
_____

What will be your first celebratory food for achieving a goal?

_____

_____

_____

_____

In this chapter, we have covered a lot of information, and I hope you have started thinking about this new journey you are starting, the journey of being healthy for life. We have discussed the key and the secret to getting to a healthy weight. We have talked about life on _Little House on the Prairie_ and how much walking they did in those days compared to now, and looked at how much we would be walking today if it were not for advances in transportation. We talked about a physical activity log, to include baseline data. Then, in section two, we talked about foods we should eat on a daily basis, eating a rainbow every day, and the nutritional values different-colored foods have.

Finally, we talked about many areas we need to include to develop a specific plan for you. Your plan needs to include the keys to weight loss, which are increased physical activity and decreased caloric intake. Additionally, we made many lists that you will have to complete and a few field trips too. I hope you will enjoy them. The field trips can be an eye-opening experience, one you will need and that will be beneficial at the start of your journey. I hope you will find some fruits and vegetables you have never eaten before that you just love. Keep in mind, some fruits and vegetables are seasonal and only available at certain times of the year, so go on field trips throughout the year. In the next chapter, we will wrap this all up, in an effort to begin our journey toward being healthy for life, a lifestyle worth having!

Chapter 6 Notes

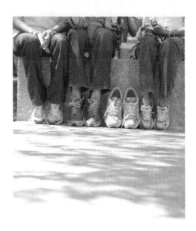

Source: jcannonphotography

DEFINITIONS

PHYSICAL ACTIVITY LOG: A log that includes all
of the physical activity you participate in for a set
period of time, similar to a reading log. You can
also include notes and goals for the set period and
keep up with achievements.

SERVING SIZE: A unit of measure used to describe
the amount of food that is recommended for each
food group. To find the recommended amount
of food, look on the Nutrition Facts or label. You

can also go to the food guide pyramid or the Dietary Guidelines for Americans.

PORTION SIZE: How much you *choose* to eat; they are as big or as small as you want them to be.

ADDITIONAL INFORMATION

Make sure before you get started you are healthy enough to participate in physical activity.

In 2009, my family started going on a 5K Turkey Trot before we eat our Thanksgiving meal. Usually, after we wake up, we have a small breakfast and get dressed. It doesn't matter how cold it is; we start on our designated journey. When we started our yearly Turkey Trots, the kids were one, three, and four years old.

My youngest son entered his first 5K when he was fourteen months old and at that point had only been walking three months. It was an Alzheimer's walk, and he was part of Team Naomi in honor of his grandma. His stroller was there as backup, but he toughed it out and walked the entire way and loved it.

A 5K (or some other walk/running event) could be a long-term goal for you to participate in. Or join me on Thanksgiving morning!

KEY POINT

The key to healthy weight is increased physical activity and decreased caloric intake or the right balance of physical activity and caloric intake.

The secret to a healthier weight is honesty!

Chapter 7: Balancing Your Scale

We have been on an enormous journey, which started by answering our first question, "What's the big deal?" I hope now, as you prepare for your next, even more enormous journey of being healthy for life, that you can answer what the big deal is regarding childhood obesity. *Today, childhood obesity is a big deal because the numbers are so high.* However, you are now equipped with the knowledge to help yourself, help family members, and help friends make the statistics not so big a deal anymore. By figuring out what your BMI is, you know not only where you are today but also how far you are from being healthy for life. Yet, more important than knowing how far you are from being healthy, you know that if you are at an unhealthy weight, you don't have to stay there and can do something to change and make positive improvements.

Years ago, I could not imagine why I would want to be physically active on a daily basis. I have always been accident prone, with the craziest incidents happening to me. I could never run well. I have asthma, tons of allergies, and a very short inseam; but sure enough, when I started my journey to healthy for life, it was physical activity that helped me reach a healthy weight and improve my health. Physical activity does not have to be running or even walking; remember, the definition of physical activity is "bodily motion resulting in energy expenditure that is produced by skeletal muscles." Physical activity can be any energy expenditure activity that you enjoy; chances are, if you enjoy it, you will participate in it more often. When physical activity is called *Miracle Gro* for the brain then it has to be pretty essential! Sixty minutes per day is not too much to aim for, considering the lifelong benefits.

It is well documented that as we get older, our level of physical fitness decreases, and this decrease is being seen in middle-school years, shortly after hitting that double-digit age. When I was in middle school, I wanted to go to college, had dreams past high school, and wanted to get old, or at least out of my teens! Physical activity and physical fitness are stepped up to a much higher level of important than ever. I hope you seriously consider how important being and staying physically active and fit are, if not for you, for those important people around you, like parents, grandparents, aunts and uncles.

Research indicates the number one reason for peer rejection in America is being overweight. I shared a story earlier, which is both heart-wrenching and scary. I cannot imagine the life that girl led, nor do I ever care for anyone to live such a life. I wonder about Manuel, and although I was only in second grade, I saw how he suffered from peer rejection. Their lives had to be a constant struggle every day; maybe they just needed a little help from someone like you who now has the tools to help.

Right now, you have the key to weight loss, and you know the secret. The key to weight loss is balancing your scale, the scale between physical activity and caloric intake, or the food and drinks you consume. The secret to weight loss is also just being honest with yourself. Without a doubt, there are hundreds of weight-loss plans out there that you can buy, but if you can just be accountable and honest to yourself, why pay for honesty? Actually, there are lots of free ones available as well. However, if you remember that one pound of fat weighs 3,500 calories and you keep up with your physical activity log and caloric intake log, then you should be on your journey to healthy for life.

I trust that you will take the information you have gained and use it positively, whether it is for you, a friend, a family member, or even someone you don't yet know, maybe a classmate. I know it may be hard, and you might start off with many excuses, like I need to see a doctor first, or my neighborhood is not safe, or I have school and a job, or I have to take care of my little brother or sister. However, remember the exercises I told you could be done inside? Remember working out at school or church before you leave? Remember weightlifting with cans at home? Life is tough, but it is much less tough when you stop making excuses and make things happen! If you cannot make things happen for the best person in the world, you, then who can you make things happen for? I know you will find a way to make things happen and make positive improvements in your life for a lifetime.

Years ago, I was an assistant principal, and I was in charge of discipline. So I saw all the crazy, wild students every day, and I had this thing—before a student left my office, I told them, "I love you!" and gave them a hug. One day after a pretty bad incident, a boy was leaving in a car that didn't belong to his parents, and due to circumstances, could not give me a hug, but before he got in the car, he turned around and, to my surprise, said, "Mrs., did you forget something?" I immediately turned around and said, "I love you!" I tell you this story to say

I care about what happens to you and hope that you listen to the information I have given you and make positive changes.

I know that sometimes parents do not have the knowledge to keep their children from becoming a statistic of childhood obesity; however, now you are equipped with the tools to help yourself and your parents. I hope you set out on your journey toward being healthy for life. The following are just a few pointers to help you get started.

- Don't try to incorporate all this the first week

- Start off with small, manageable goals

- Set goals, schedules, and deadlines

- Add nutritious food whenever you can

- Eat breakfast every morning

- Limit red meat consumption

- Try some fish, chicken, or turkey

- Make a game out of exercising

- Add a little competition

- Make a weekly menu

- Drink some milk

- Write down monthly goals

  Good luck, and I wish you the best!

A Final Word

There are a few different ways you can use this book, all of which I hope benefit you in some way, along with any friends or relatives you might be trying to help. You could be reading this book:

- because you do not want to become a childhood obesity statistic;

- because you are obese and want to make positive changes in your life; or

- because you want to help a friend or family member make positive changes in his or her life.

At this point, I hope that you are still with me; but in addition, I hope you have learned at least a few things, enjoyed a few stories, been touched by something, and are ready to start your new journey. As a parent, one of the most shocking pieces of research I found when I started my journey learning about childhood obesity was that for the first time in this country, parents are burying their children at very young ages due to complications caused by childhood obesity. A very special

Papaw once told me no parent should ever have to endure the pain of burying a child. When I read the same shocking information as an educator, I thought I *had* to do something. I could not simply continue to learn about this problem without attempting to help the very people suffering. As a teacher and former parent educator, I knew what I needed to do. I needed to talk directly to the people suffering, not the parents, because there is that possibility that parents are also overweight or obese and may not know how to lead either you or themselves on a journey toward being healthy for life.

As I stated in the book, the key to a healthy weight is balancing your physical activity with your caloric intake. Therefore, to start your journey toward healthy for life, you first need to know how much physical activity you engage in and how many calories you consume on a daily basis. Once you determine this, you can start to balance your scale. The physical activity log and the caloric intake log will be great tools for you in determining the answers to both questions (and they are free). Additionally, the tools may be simple and easily replicated but tools you can use for years to come in an effort to stay on the right path toward your journey of healthy for life. You can also share them with others.

Lots of luck to you.

And never forget, the secret is honesty!

Afterword

Upon writing this book, I had four goals for you, the reader:

- You will better understand the big picture of what childhood obesity is, including research, statistics, what it all means, and how it may relate to you.

- You will learn how *not* to be included in these statistics.

- You will learn to live a life full of good health, free of ailments caused by obesity.

- You can share the information and knowledge you gain by reading this book with others.

After having read this far, I hope I was successful in at least a few, if not all of these goals. I hope this book has given you the information and tools you were looking for to become healthy for life. When you think about this journey, I hope you realize that being healthy for life is actually a lifestyle, not a diet or fad. In order to maintain a balanced scale (physical activity and caloric intake), you will have to make physical activity and eating healthy part of your life *every day.*

Now, please do not think you have to calculate your physical activity and determine your caloric intake every day for the rest of your life. Luckily for us all, the more you keep up with it, the easier it gets, and it becomes second nature. I will say there have been times when I don't calculate my caloric intake, such as when I travel, a day or two during the holidays, and recently when I was "homeless" for a month. Not being in a place where you can weigh and measure your food, plus being at the mercy of having to eat out for an extended period of time do present problems, but stick to what you know to be healthy. Also, stay physically active during times that present a problem for you, so you don't have to worry as much when you get back to your routine. In addition, try to plan for those times when you know you are going to have that delicious banana pudding Vivian made or when you will be going to the big Vaca barbeque or fish fry. This can be done by eating fewer calories on the days before and after and participating in extra physical activity, in an attempt to make up for the splurge. *Always* plan to get back on track as soon as possible, typically the next day.

When I first started my journey, I wasn't seeing results too fast and obviously wanted results immediately. My Daddy always said, "Anything worth having is worth working hard for." Therefore, the more I worked, the harder I worked, I finally started seeing positive results. After all, I didn't get unhealthy and overweight overnight—so be patient, but be persistent. *It will happen!*

Conclusion

I wrote this book to give you the knowledge and tools you need to be healthy for life! This is not a diet, it is a lifestyle; the difference is, diets are for a certain period of time. They come and go and many change often. Others do not practice the secret to a healthy weight, and it seems they are on a diet most of their life, unsuccessfully attempting to lose weight. A lifestyle is how you live every day. Thus, if you plan on living healthy once in a while, just start the next new diet craze. But if you plan on living a healthy life forever, keep your scale balanced. I realize while you are on your journey, there will be times when you hop off the healthy-for-life path to pick up a plate of barbeque or attend a fish fry, just like I do at times. Being prepared for those times and getting back on your journey as soon as possible will keep you healthy for life!

Good luck on your journey, stay strong, and Godspeed.

About the Author

A first-time author, Olga worked in education for fourteen years, in both elementary and secondary, as well as in school and district administration. She has degrees in elementary and special education, educational administration, and a doctorate in educational leadership, with specializations in early childhood, bilingual education, and educational diagnostics. She is currently working on a journal to complement her book and a second book, which will also be about childhood obesity, but will be a resource for parents. Currently Olga finds herself juggling the arduous tasks of being a military wife, mother of three young, very active children, and her journey toward being healthy for life. Olga, her husband, and children call Texas home, however, the military takes them on many adventures.

Appendices

2007 - 2008 Data FITNESSGRAM® Data
(% Achieving Healthy Fitness Zone on all 6

Grade	Total # Tested	Girls (%)	Boys (%)
3	102,342	33.25	28.6
4	80,539	28.5	21.14
5	66,798	23.82	17.89
6	60,663	23.08	17.6
7	55,441	21.32	17.26
8	48,971	18.99	17.88
9	39,456	13.9	15.04
10	28,650	12.42	13.7
11	21,152	10.68	12.24
12	13,040	8.18	8.96

Students Assessed: 2,658,665
Districts Submitting: 1,074 (84.77%)

2008 - 2009 Data FITNESSGRAM® Data
(% Achieving Healthy Fitness Zone on all 6

Grade	Total # Tested	Girls (%)	Boys (%)
3	116,096	36.42	30.89
4	95,842	33.53	24.55
5	79,281	28.02	20.85
6	75,610	28.2	20.55
7	66,950	26.01	19.58
8	60,004	22.28	19.8
9	46,206	16.25	16.14
10	32,865	13.33	13.88
11	24,416	11.1	12.16
12	15,468	8.78	9.25

Students Assessed: 2,801,486
Districts Submitting: 1,132 (89.42%)

2009 - 2010 Data FITNESSGRAM® Data
(% Achieving Healthy Fitness Zone on all 6

Grade	Total # Tested	Girls (%)	Boys (%)
3	119,401	37.27	30.98
4	102,709	34.22	25.26
5	87,389	30.12	21.81
6	83,982	30.23	27.7
7	76,555	28.14	21.42
8	67,218	24.18	21.62
9	48,278	17.04	15.71
10	32,069	13.16	12.98
11	23,431	10.6	11.14
12	15,214	8.07	8.54

Students Assessed: 2,903,200
Districts Submitting: 1,141 (92.24%)

Source: TEA

Physical Activity Log:

Physical Activity Log for (week):							Notes:			
Sun.	Mon.	Tues.	Wed.	Thurs.	Fri.	Sat.				

GOALS	ACHIEVED
1.) Work out four days per week	
2.) Work out at least twenty minutes each time	
3.) Try thirty minutes at least once	

Caloric Intake Log

Sun.	Mon.	Tues.	Wed.
B-fast: _____	B-fast: _____	B-fast: _____	B-fast: _____
Snack: _____	Snack: _____	Snack: _____	Snack: _____
Lunch: _____	Lunch: _____	Lunch: _____	Lunch: _____
Snack: _____	Snack: _____	Snack: _____	Snack: _____
Dinner: _____	Dinner: _____	Dinner: _____	Dinner: _____
Snack: _____	Snack: _____	Snack: _____	Snack: _____
TOTAL: _____	*TOTAL:* _____	*TOTAL:* _____	*TOTAL:* _____

153

Thurs.	Fri.	Sat.	Notes:
B-fast: _____	B-fast: _____	B-fast: _____	_____
Snack: _____	Snack: _____	Snack: _____	_____
Lunch: _____	Lunch: _____	Lunch: _____	_____
Snack: _____	Snack: _____	Snack: _____	_____
Dinner: _____	Dinner: _____	Dinner: _____	_____
Snack: _____	Snack: _____	Snack: _____	_____
TOTAL: _____	TOTAL: _____	TOTAL: _____	

My Exercise Chart

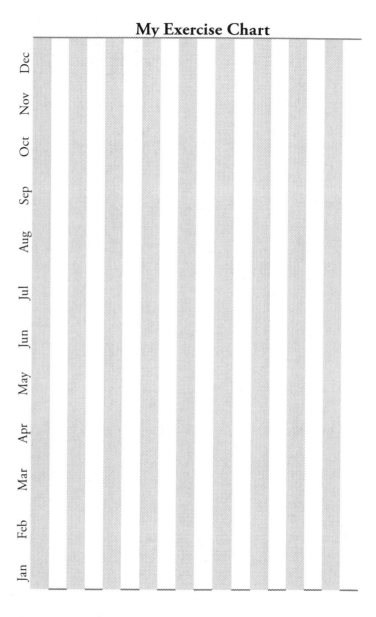

Date

Jan Feb Mar Apr May Jun Jul Aug Sep Oct Nov Dec

1 2 3 4 5 6 7 8 9 10 11 12 13 14 15 16 17 18

Date	Jan	Feb	Mar	Apr	May	Jun	Jul	Aug	Sep	Oct	Nov	Dec
19												
20												
21												
22												
23												
24												
25												
26												
27												
28												
29												
30												
31												
TOTAL												
S												
B												
H												
A												

G l o s s a r y

Body mass index (BMI) – a reliable indicator of body fatness for most children and teens. It is calculated according to a child's weight and height and is age- and sex-specific for children and teens. The formula to calculate BMI is as follows: weight (pounds) / height (inches)^2 x 703. A BMI includes the following weight-status categories at the specified percentile ranges (Centers for Disease Control and Prevention, 2010): underweight—less than the fifth percentile; healthy weight—fifth percentile to less than the eighty-fifth percentile; overweight—eighty-fifth to less than the ninety-fifth percentile; and obese—equal to or greater than the ninety-fifth percentile.

Caloric Intake – calories that are consumed.

Exercise – a subset of physical activity that is planned, structured, and repetitive. Its purpose is to improve or maintain physical fitness.

Fitnessgram – an assessment created in 1982 by The Cooper Institute of Dallas, which measures the following fitness areas in students: body composition; aerobic capacity; and strength, endurance, and flexibility.

Globesity – the global epidemic of obesity or how obesity is affecting so many countries throughout the world.

Healthy Fitness Zone (HFZ) – a criterion-referenced standard, based on levels of fitness needed for good health, set specifically for boys and girls of various ages; not based on class averages or peer comparisons.

Kinesiology – the study of the mechanics of body movements.

Obesity – a term the Centers for Disease Control stated is two categories above a healthy weight range and includes a body mass index (BMI) of 30 or more.

Pediatric exercise science – the study of exercise during childhood.

Physical activity – bodily motion resulting in energy expenditure that is produced by skeletal muscles.

Physical fitness – a subset of exercises that are either health- or skill-related.

Portion size – how much you choose to eat, during either a meal or snack, so a portion is as big or as small as you want it to be.

Sedentary activities – activities involving sitting and correspondingly little motion or exercise.

Self-esteem – thinking that you are important or valuable. It is not that you think you are perfect and better than everyone else. It is more like thinking you are worthy of being loved and accepted.

Serving size – a fixed amount of food, such as one cup or one ounce, shown on the Nutrition Facts label. It is useful in determining how much of that particular food you eat and what amount of nutrients you are getting, and in making comparisons among foods.

Sleep apnea – a common disorder in which you have one or more pauses in breathing or shallow breaths while you sleep. Breathing pauses can last from a few seconds to minutes. They often occur five to thirty times or more an hour. Typically, normal breathing then starts again, sometimes with a loud snort or choking sound. Sleep apnea usually is a chronic (ongoing) condition that disrupts your sleep. You often move out of deep sleep and into light sleep when your breathing pauses or becomes shallow. The most common type of sleep apnea is obstructive sleep apnea, meaning the airway has collapsed or is blocked during sleep, which may cause shallow breathing or breathing pauses. Obstructive sleep apnea is more common in people who are overweight but can affect anyone; for example, small children may have enlarged tonsil tissues in their throats, which can lead to obstructive sleep apnea.

Type-II diabetes – a form of diabetes that usually occurs in people over forty years of age but may develop in younger people, especially in minorities. Most people who develop type-II diabetes are insulin-resistant. However, some simply cannot produce enough insulin to meet their body's needs, and others have a combination of these problems. Many people with type-II diabetes control the disease through diet and exercise, but some must also take oral medications or insulin.

Resources

American Cancer Society

http://www.cancer.org/

American Diabetes Services

http://www.americandiabetes.com/

American Heart Association

http://www.heart.org/HEARTORG/

Be Active, Healthy, and Happy! 2008 Physical Activity
Guidelines for Americans by the US Department of

Health and Human Services

http://www.health.gov/paguidelines/guidelines/default.aspx

BMI Percentile Calculator for Child and Teen, Centers for
Disease Control and Prevention

http://apps.nccd.cdc.gov/dnpabmi/

Centers for Disease Control and Prevention

http://www.cdc.gov/

Centers for Disease Control and Prevention, Fruits and Veggies More Matters

http://www.fruitsandveggiesmatter.gov/

Cooper Institute, The

http://www.cooperinstitute.org/

Dietary Guidelines for Americans 2010, booklet, by US Department of Agriculture and US Department of Health and Human Services

http://health.gov/dietaryguidelines/dga2010/DietaryGuidelines2010.pdf

Fitnessgram

http://www.fitnessgram.net/home/

Kids' Health

http://kidshealth.org/kid/

Let's Move, America's Move to Raise a Healthier Generation of Kids

http://www.letsmove.gov/

Media-Smart Youth: Eat, Think, and Be Active. National Institutes of Health, Eunice Kennedy Shriver,

National Institute of Child Health and Human Development

http://www.nichd.nih.gov/msy/

National Cancer Institute at the National Institutes of Health

http://www.cancer.gov/

National Football League, Play 60

http://www.nfl.com/play60

National Institutes of Health, Eunice Kennedy Shriver, National Institute of Child Health & Human Development

http://www.nichd.nih.gov/milk/milk.cfm

Navy Operational Fueling, by the US Department of the Navy

http://www.cnrc.navy.mil/noru/html/downloads/NOFFS_Nutrition.pdf

President's Challenge, The

https://www.presidentschallenge.org/

Take Charge of Your Health, by United States Department of Health and Human Services

http://win.niddk.nih.gov/publications/PDFs/teenblackwhite3.pdf

Trust for America's Health, Preventing Epidemics, Protecting People

http://healthyamericans.org/

United States Department of Agriculture, Centers for Nutrition Policy and Promotion

http://www.cnpp.usda.gov/

United States Department of Agriculture, Food and Nutrition Service website

http://teamnutrition.usda.gov/Default.htm

United States Department of Agriculture, Know Your Farmer, Know Your Food

http://www.usda.gov/wps/portal/usda/knowyourfarmer?na vid=KNOWYOURFARMER

United States Department of Agriculture, My Plate.gov

http://www.choosemyplate.gov/

United States Department of Agriculture, The People's Garden

http://www.usda.gov/wps/portal/usda/ usdahome?navid=PEOPLES_GARDEN

United States Department of Health and Human Services

http://www.nih.gov/

United States Department of Health and Human Services, Deliciously Healthy Eating (includes various healthy eating recipes)

http://hp2010.nhlbihin.net/healthyeating/default.aspx

United States Department of Health and Human Services, National Institute of Diabetes and Digestive and Kidney Diseases

http://www2.niddk.nih.gov/

United States Department of Health and Human Services, US Food and Drug Administration

http://www.fda.gov/

References

American Association for the Advancement of Science (2006). *Obesity: The science inside*. Washington, D. C.

American Public Health Association (2012). *Direct causes: Too much food, too little physical activity*. Retrieved frm http://www.apha.org/programs/resources/obesity/obesityrootdirect.htm.

Baranowski, T., Cullen, K. W., Nicklas, T., Thompson, D., and Baranoski, J. (2003). "Are current health behavioral change models helpful in guiding prevention of weight gain efforts?" *Obesity Research*, 11, 23S–43S.

Beighle, A., Pangrazi, R. P., & Vincent, S. D. (2001). Pedometers, physical activity and accountability. *Journal of Physical Education, Recreation & Dance*, 72(9), 16-36.

Black, M. H., Smith, N., Porter, A. H., Jacobsen, S. J., & Koebnick, C. (2010). Higher prevalence of obesity among children with asthma. *Obesity* 20(5) 1041-1047.

Brittenham, S. W. and Reed, J. A. (2004). "Physical activity and physical fitness: What is the difference?" *South Carolina Journal of Health, Physical Education, Recreation and Dance*, 34 (1), 36–39.

Bryan, M. (2006). "Obesity in America and its impact on minorities, women and low-income groups." *International Journal of the Diversity*, 6 (3), 97–101.

California Department of Education (2002). *State study proves physically fit kids perform better academically.* Retrieved from *http://www.cahperd.org/images/pdf_docs/CDE_News_Release.pdf.*

Campbell, K. (2007). "Why is everyone going on about childhood overweight and what can we do about it?" *Nutridate*, 18 (1), 1–5.

Carlson, S. A., Fulton, J. E., Lee, S. M., Maynard, L. M., Brown, D. R., Kohl, III, H. W., and Dietz, W. H. (2008). "Physical education and academic achievement in elementary school: Data from the early childhood longitudinal study." *American Journal of Public Health*, 98 (4), 721–727.

Centers for Disease Control and Prevention (2011). *National diabetes fact sheet: national estimates and general information on diabetes and prediabetes in the United States, 2011.* Retrieved from http://www.cdc.gov/diabetes/pubs/pdf/ndfs_2011.pdf.

Centers for Disease Control and Prevention, National Center for Environmental Health, Division of Environmental Hazards and Health Effects (2011). *CDC vital signs, asthma in the US growing every year.* Retrieved from http://www.cdc.gov/VitalSigns/pdf/2011-05-vitalsigns.pdf.

Centers for Disease Control and Prevention (2010). *Childhood overweight and obesity.* Retrieved from *http://www.cdc.gov/obesity/childhood/index.html.*

Chomitz, V. R., Slining, M. M., McGowan, R. J., Mitchell, S. E., Dawson, G. F., and Hacker, K. A. (2009). "Is there a relationship between physical fitness and academic achievement? Positive results from public school children in the northeastern United States." *Journal of School Health,* 79 (1), 30–37.

Cook, G. (2005). "Killing PE is killing our kids the slow way." *American School Board Journal,* 192, 16–19.

Cooper Institute, The (2008). *Fitness of Texas students shocking.* Retrieved from *http://www.cooperinstitute.org/ourkidshealth/news/documents/Summer _OpEd.pdf.*

_____. (2009). *Summary of Texas youth fitness study initial results.* Retrieved from *http://www.cooperinstitute.org/ourkidshealth/documents /Texas%20Youth%20Fitness%20Study%20--%20Chart.pdf.*

_____. (2009). *The obesity epidemic in children—An alarming trend.* Retrieved from *http://cooperinstitute.org/ourkidshealth/documents /Texas.*

Creswell, J. W. (2008). *Educational research, planning, conducting, and evaluating quantitative and qualitative research.* Upper Saddle River, NJ: Pearson prentice Hall.

Datar, A., Sturm, R., and Magnabosco, J. L. (2004). "Childhood overweight and academic performance: National study of kindergartners and first-graders." *Obesity Research,* 12 (1), 58–68.

Ehrlich, G. (2008). "Health = performance, efforts to increase student achievement also should address physical activity and a good diet." *American School Board Journal,* 195 (10), 42–44.

Ganz, M. L. (2003). "The economic evaluation of obesity interventions: Its time has come." *Obesity Research,* 11 (11), 1275–1277.

Goel, M. S., McCarthy, E. P., Phillips, R. S., and Wee, C. C. (2004). "Obesity among US immigrant subgroups by duration of residence." *Journal of the American Medical Association,* 292 (23), 2860–2867.

Human Kinetics (2008). *Fitnessgram/activitygram, activity and fitness assessment, reporting, and tracking—the most valid and reliable tool available* [brochure]. LC: Author.

_____. (2008). *Fitnessgram/activitygram overview.* Retrieved from *http://www.fitnessgram.net/home/.*

Malecka-Tendera E., and Mazur, A. (2006). "Childhood obesity: A pandemic of the twenty-first century." *International Journal of Obesity,* 30 (S), 1–3.

Malik, V. S., Schulze, M. B., & Hu, F. B. (2006). "Intake of sugar-sweetened beverages and weight gain: A systematic review [1-3]." *American Journal of Clinical Nutrition,* 84, 274-288.

Martin, L., and Chalmers, G. (2007). "The relationship between academic achievement and physical fitness." *Physical Educator,* 64 (4), 214–221.

National Association for Sport and Physical Education (2002). *New study proves physically fit kids perform better academically*. Retrieved from *http://www.aahperd.org/naspe/template.cfm?template=pr_121002.html*.

National Education Association (1999). Report on size discrimination. Washington, D. C.

Ogden, C. L., Carroll, M., Curtin, L., Lamb, M., and Flegal, K. (2010). "Prevalence of high body mass index in US children and adolescents 2007–2008." *Journal of American Medical Association*, 303 (3), 242–249.

Pangrazi, R. P., and Corbin, C. B. (1990). "Age as a factor relating to physical fitness test performance." *Research Quarterly for Exercise and Sport*, 61 (4), 410–414.

Prosser, L., and Jiang, X. (2008). "Relationship between school physical activity and academic performance of children." *The International Journal of Learning*, 15 (3), 11–16.

Pyle, S. A., Sharkey, J., Yetter, G., Felix, E., Furlong, M. J., and Poston, W. S. (2006). "Fighting an epidemic: The role of schools in reducing childhood obesity." *Psychology in the Schools*, 43 (3), 361–376.

Reed, J., Brittenham, S., Phillips, D., and Carlisle, C. (2007). "A preliminary examination of the fitness levels of children who meet the president's council physical activity recommendation." *Physical Educator*, 64 (3), 159–167.

Robert Wood Johnson Foundation (2007). *Active education, physical education, physical activity and academic performance. Research brief*, 1–4.

Schumacher, D., and Queen, J. A. (2007). *Overcoming obesity in childhood and adolescence, A guide for school leaders.* Thousand Oaks, CA: Corwin Press.

Schwimmer, J. B., Burwinkle, T. M., & Varni, J. W., (2003). Health-related quality of life of severely obese children and adolescents. *Journal of American Medical Association,* 289 (14), 1813-1819.

Sibley, B. A., and Ward, R. M. (2008). "Making the grade with diet and exercise." *AASA Journal of Scholarship and Practice,* 5 (2), 38–45.

Small, L., Anderson, D., and Mazurek Melnyk, B., (2007). "Prevention and early treatment of overweight and obesity in young children: A critical review and appraisal of the evidence." *Pediatric Nursing,* 33 (2), 149–161.

Society of State Directors of Health, Physical Education and Recreation. (2005). *Resolution for quality physical education and physical activity.* Adopted October 18, 2005.

Spiegel, S. A., and Foulk, D. (2006). "Reducing overweight through a multidisciplinary school-based intervention." *Obesity,* 14 (1), 88–96.

Stegelin, D. A. (2008). "Children, teachers, and families working together to prevent childhood obesity: Intervention strategies." *Dimensions of Early Childhood,* 36 (1), 8–15.

Strauss, R. S. (2000). "Childhood obesity and self-esteem." *Pediatrics,* 105 (1)e15.

Taras, H. (2005). "Physical activity and student performance at school." *Journal of School Health,* 75 (6), 214–218.

Taras, H., and Potts–Datema, W. (2005). "Obesity and student performance at school." *Journal of School Health*, 75 (8), 291–295.

Texas Education Agency (2002). "State board of education approves mandatory physical activity program for K–6 students." *Texas Education Today*, XV (4), 2.

_____ (2003). *Timeline of testing in Texas.* Retrieved from *http://ritter.tea.state.tx.us/student.assessment/resources/studies/testingtimeline.pdf.*

_____ (2008). *Texas tests fitness of 2.6 million students: Finds elementary students are in best shape.* Retrieved from *http://www.tea.state.tx.us/press/08fitnessresults.pdf#xml=http://www.tea.state.tx.us/cgi/texis/webinator/search/xml.txt?query=Texas+tests+fitness+of+2.6+million+students%3B+finds+elementary+students+are+in+best+shape&db=db&id=c8a07ae26cf02cc8.*

_____ (2009). *Physically fit students more likely to do well in school, less likely to be disciplinary problems.* Retrieved from *http://cooperinstitute.org/ourkidshealth/documents/fitnessresults09.pdf.*

Texas Legislature (2007). *Senate bill 530–Bill Text.* Retrieved from *http://www.legis.state.tx.us/tlodocs/80R/billtext/html/SB00530F.htm.*

Trachtenberg, J. (2007). *The real age guide to raising healthy children, good kids bad habits.* New York, NY: Harper Collins Publishers.

Trost, S. G., and van der Mars, H. (2010). "Why we should not cut P.E." *Educational Leadership*, 67 (4), 60–65.

Trost, S. G. (2007). *Physical education, physical activity and academic performance.* Princeton, NJ: The Robert Wood Johnson Foundation.

Trust for America's Health (2007). *State data: Obesity rates, % children age 10-17.* Retrieved from http://healthyamericans. org/states/states.php?measure=overwieght&sort=data.

US Department of Health and Human Services (2008). *2008 Physical activity guidelines for Americans.* Retrieved from *www.health.gov/paguidelines.*

US Department of Health and Human Services, Centers for Disease Control Prevention (2007). *What is body mass index?* Retrieved from *http://www.cdc.gov/nccdphp/dnpa/ bmi/adult_BMI/about_adult_BMI.htm.*

US Department of Health and Human Services, Centers for Disease Control and Prevention, National Centers for Chronic Disease Prevention and Health Promotion, and The President's Council on Physical Fitness and Sports (1999). *Physical activity and health, a report of the surgeon general executive summary.* Retrieved from *www.cdc. gov/needphp/sgr/contents.htm.*

US Department of Health and Human Services, National Institutes of Health (2009). *Portion Distortion.* Retrieved from *http://hp2010.nhlbihin.net/portion/index.htm.*

US Department of Health and Human Services, Centers for Disease Control and Prevention (2010). *Health, United States, 2010, with special feature on death and dying.* Retrieved from http://www.cdc.gov/nchs/data/hus/hus10.pdf.

US Department of the Navy (2010). *Navy Operational Fueling*. Retrieved from *http://www.cnrc.navy.mil/noru/html/downloads/NOFFS_Nutrition.pdf*.

US House of Representatives, Committee on Education and Labor (2008). *Improving physical education in US schools is key to fighting child obesity epidemic, witnesses tell house education committee*. Press Release July 24, 2008.

Vaca Durr, O. A. (2010). "The Relationship between Physical Fitness and Academic Achievement in Math and Science in a Select Texas School District." Unpublished doctoral dissertation, University of Mary Hardin Baylor, Belton, Texas.

Vail, K. (2006). "Mind and body, new research ties physical activity and fitness to academic success." *American School Board Journal*, 193 (3), 330–333.

Welk, G. J. and Meredith, M. D. (Eds.) (2008). *Fitnessgram/Activitygram Reference Guide*. Dallas, TX: The Cooper Institute.

White House Task Force on Childhood Obesity. (2010). *Solving the problem of childhood obesity within a generation, White House task force on childhood obesity report to the president*. Retrieved from *http://www.letsmove.gov/tfco_fullreport_may2010.pdf*.

Yu, C. C. W., Chan, S., Cheng, F., Sung, R. Y. T., and Hau, K. T. (2006). "Are physical activity and academic performance compatible? Academic achievement, conduct, physical activity and self–esteem of Hong Kong Chinese primary school children." *Educational Studies*, 32 (4), 331–341.

Index

Nutrition Fact 107

W